THE
Stay **Strong** Mummy
FITNESS PLAN

THE
Stay **Strong** Mummy
FITNESS PLAN

KIMBERLEY WELMAN WITH VICTORIA REIHANA

piatkus

PIATKUS

First published in Great Britain in 2017 by Piatkus
1 3 5 7 9 10 8 6 4 2

A CIP catalogue record for this book
is available from the British Library.

ISBN 978-0-349-41421-8

Recipe photography © Ellen De Meulemeester
Lifestyle photography © Kit Wise
Designed by D.R. ink
Edited by Jan Cutler
Printed and bound in China by C&C Offset Printing Co, Ltd

Papers used by Piatkus are from well managed
forests and other responsible sources

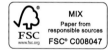

Piatkus
An imprint of
Little, Brown Book Group
Carmelite House
50 Victoria Embankment
London EC4Y 0DZ

An Hachette UK Company
www.hachette.co.uk

www.improvementzone.co.uk

Disclaimer
The dietary information and exercises in this book are not intended to replace or conflict with the
advice given to you by your GP or other health professionals. All matters regarding your health
should be discussed with your GP. The authors and publisher disclaim any liability directly or
indirectly from the use of the material in this book by any person.

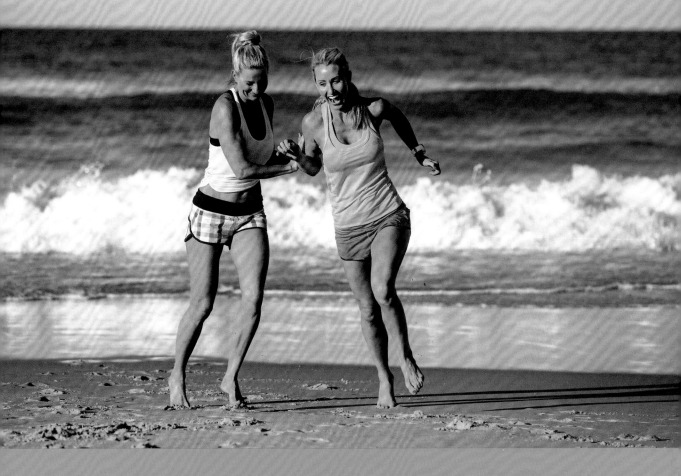

This book was written for mummies
all over the world – to help you to believe
in your strength and beauty

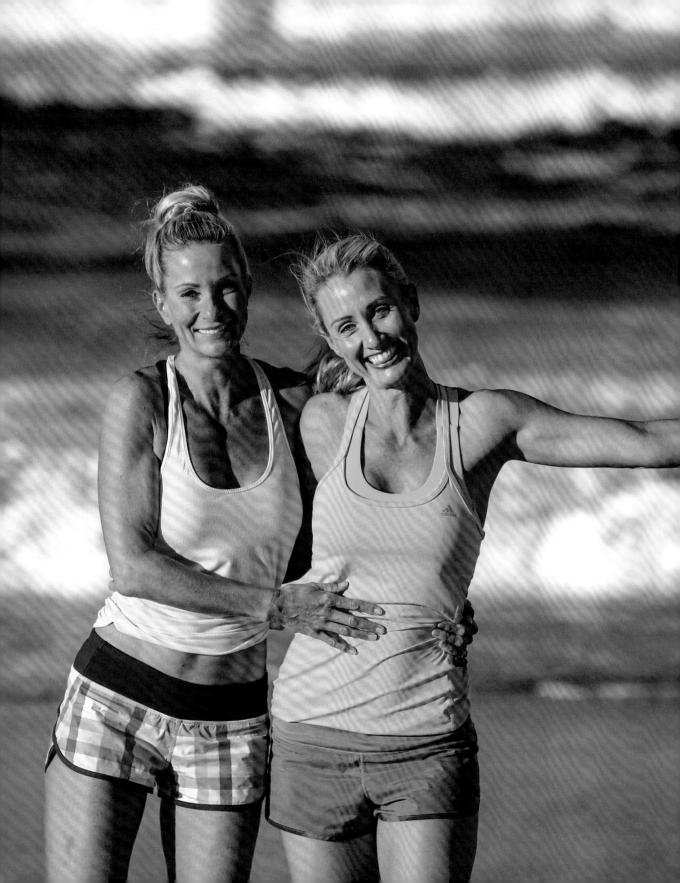

About the Authors

Kimberley Welman

Kimberley enjoyed four years as a stay-at-home mother before returning to work to manage her online parents' support forum and blog *StayStrongMummy*, as well as working as a consultant to various businesses as a social and digital communications manager. With three children born within 19 months, Kimberley knows first hand that life as a parent definitely isn't always rainbows, butterflies, squats and baby chinos. And because she's lived it, she dedicates her life to empowering other mums to be the best they can be, in fitness, health and happiness.

This inspiring mum takes all that she's learned from being a parent and helps others to realise that it's how you pick yourself up, brush yourself off and get moving that makes the world of difference to a healthy, happy family.

Prior to having children, Kimberley enjoyed a 12-year career as a senior public relations consultant for one of Australia's longest-serving corporate communication firms. Her background in media, interviews, broadcast TV, event management, press conferences, strategy management and reporting has played an integral role in the success of her blog and social media pages.

In the span of just two years, Kimberley has gained a loyal social media following of over 100,000. She connects with her audience every week via her social media channels and website.

Victoria Reihana

Vicky Reihana is a mum of two, an entrepreneur and a certified holistic health coach. She completed her studies under the Institute of Integrative Nutrition, one of the world's largest nutrition school and certification programs. Vicky also holds a certification in Fitness and Personal Training, and is the founder of a natural superfood protein blend. In addition, she is certified in Metabolic Precision Body Transformation System, Science-based Prescription for Muscle Building, Australian KettleBell Training and is also an RPM (bike) instructor.

Vicky's passion lies in holistic health and nutrition, and she has become renowned for wowing some of the world's top athletes and wholefood bloggers with her unique approach to nutrition and exercise.

She loves to inspire others and is determined to show the world how being fit and healthy are the keys to a balanced, happy and fulfilling life. Fittingly, Vicky's radiance is a testament not only to her vitality but to her healthy living and way of life.

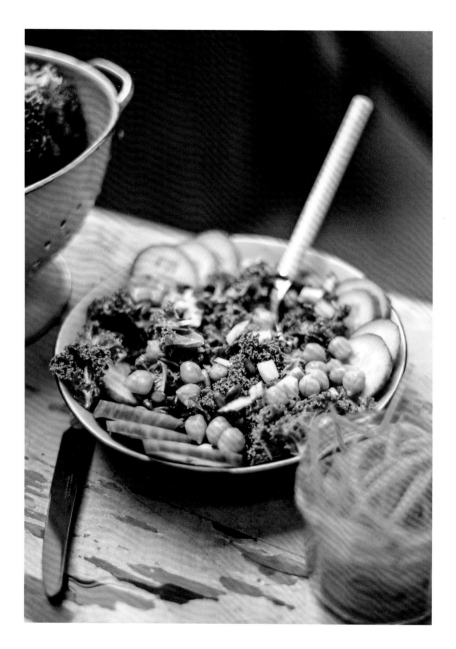

CONTENTS

Acknowledgements

They say it takes a village to raise a child. We believe it also takes a village to raise a mother. We wouldn't have been able to write this book without the tremendous amount of support, encouragement and love that we have received from our families, friends and social media tribe. *The Stay Strong Mummy Fitness Plan* isn't just about sharing our health and fitness journey – it's an in-depth reflection on our lives as mothers. Every word reflects an experience, conversation, meal, workout or heartfelt moment from within the walls of our own homes. We've shared plenty of laughs and joyous moments working on this book, but we've also shed tears, gone through tireless all-nighters on the computer and had intense moments of fear and self-doubt. To see this book in its entirety and in the hands of women around the world will forever be one of life's most memorable moments.

Thank you to our literary agent Mackenzie Brady for believing in us and giving us the confidence to fulfil our dream, and to our amazing publishers at Little, Brown in the UK for taking our dream and turning it into a reality. Thank you to our own mummies for their endless support, love and guidance; to our families for surrounding us with a beam of light, love, laughter and encouragement; and to our children, for showing us what endless love is all about – you are, by far, our greatest and proudest achievements. And, to our husbands – the men who radiate a sense of strength, love and security in all that they do and who still, to this day, make our hearts skip a beat when they walk in the door each day – thank you for arming us with the self-belief to do this.

This book is dedicated to every family in the world. Never underestimate the healing powers of a real, home-cooked meal, gentle exercise, laughing around the dinner table and just being together.

Special note by Kimberley: This book is also written in honour of my late father, Werner Joseph Hrastovec. While you never got to meet your grandchildren, we see you in their eyes every day. Thank you for giving me the confidence to be a leader.

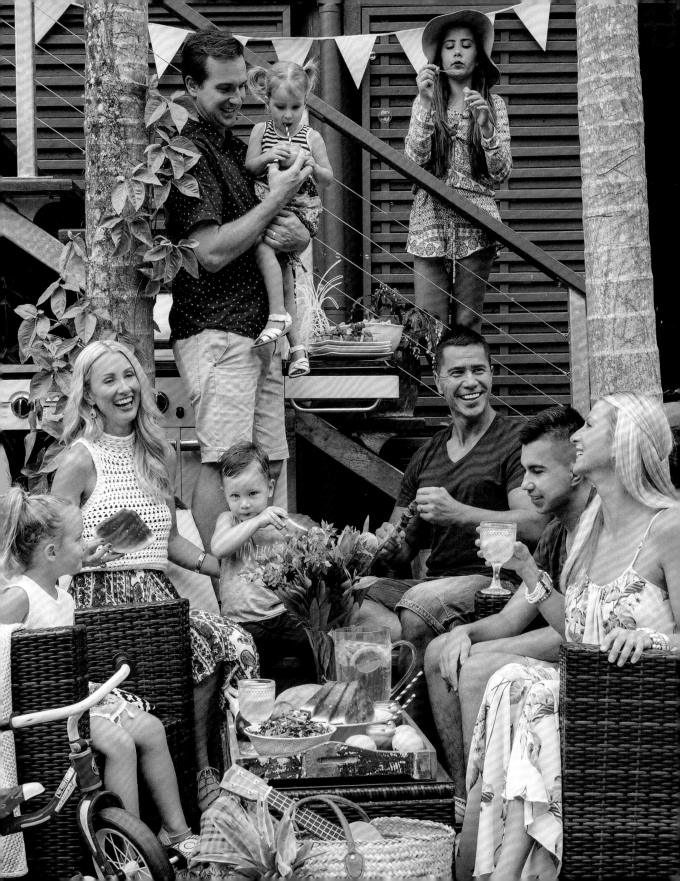

Introduction

Welcome, darling mumma! We're so thrilled that this book has landed in your hands and that you're feeling the pull to live a healthier, happier, fitter and stronger life as a mother. Stay Strong Mummy is our gift to you, to help you be the very best mum you can – and, of course, to help you to feel vibrant and bursting with vitality. This book has every bit of info you'll need to be healthy, happy and fit. We're here for you, because we know how important being a mum is to you and because we want you to realise just how important you are too.

Motherhood is an absolute gift, but it can also be an emotional rollercoaster ride. One minute you can be dancing with joy in the living room and the next minute you're reduced to tears, feeling completely and utterly exhausted.

Being a mum takes you on an incredible journey that brings new meaning to life and opens up your heart and mind. It fills your love cup in a way that you never thought possible. It is also true, however, that being a parent can soak up every ounce of your energy, leaving you feeling uncertain of yourself, isolated and sometimes stark raving crazy. It's easy to get lost in motherhood – lost in the chores, lost in the errands, lost in busy schedules, lost in our minds, lost in our relationships and lost in ourselves. That's one of the reasons why we started documenting our own personal journeys, and that's why Stay Strong Mummy was created. We wanted to create a special space where mothers could unite, support each other and gain an insight into the foundations that have helped us on our own motherhood journeys. And now it's time for us to share our hard-earned wisdom with you – so that you can really rock this motherhood thing!

'Motherhood is an absolute gift, but it can also be an emotional rollercoaster ride'

The title of this book, *The Stay Strong Mummy Fitness Plan*, embodies the importance of finding and maintaining your strength, both physically and emotionally. Physical strength is super-important for women as we age – because being physically strong helps with increased energy, fitness, bone density, skin elasticity, toning and weight loss. Emotional strength is equally important; it's about being kinder to yourself and loving the skin you're in. Self-acceptance and being able to nourish the beautiful woman within can easily become a lost art once we have kids, so Stay Strong Mummy was created to help you reclaim your strength and give you the knowledge, skills and courage to get super-strong and, at the same time, love who you really are. Physical and emotional strength always work hand in hand, and you do need to pay attention to both elements of strength in order to reap the benefits of a healthy, vibrant life.

Vicky: Our 'why'

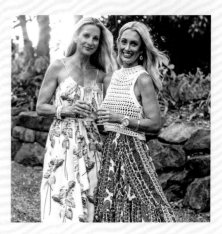

With so much conflicting information available on health, weight loss and fitness, many people are left confused about the basics of a healthy diet and a maintainable exercise regime. Because we know how tricky it can be to find the right advice when it comes to health and fitness for mums, we decided to be proactive and craft a book specifically designed to help you cut through all the noise – to give busy mums, just like you and me, the essential tools they need to enhance their fitness, health and happiness. So, here it is: Stay Strong Mummy will be your guide to healthy eating, fitness and well-being, and all the other stuff that goes into helping you be the very best mummy you can be.

Our workouts can be performed in the comfort of your own home – or even on the go – with little to no equipment (kids make great weights!), and our nutritional plan is achievable on a tight budget. You won't need to be a master chef, either.

We have aimed to provide you with a cost- and time-effective solution to health, fitness and personal success. We are two busy mothers, just like you, who have combined parenting experience of over 20 years. Kimberley and I offer different perspectives, experiences and hard-earned wisdom – and, perhaps most importantly, we get what it's like to be a mum. It is our greatest wish that every mum who picks this book up will take on board a valuable life-changing lesson and have the support, courage and determination to use it to better their lives and the lives of those they love. There really is something in this book for every mum, regardless of age, culture, financial status or lifestyle, and we know that there's something in here for you too.

Together, Kimberley and I challenge you, as you digest the words of wisdom and delicious recipes within this book, to look a little deeper into yourself and to break through any emotional barriers that have been holding you back. We want you to use this book as a reference to explore and fulfil a life of educated, healthy living, clean eating and a fitter, happier you.

A mother's time with her children is so precious. That's what makes the Stay Strong Mummy Plan so perfect for you and your little ones. What could be more convenient and better suited to family life than 15-minute workouts and easy-peasy, quick and nutritious family meals?

Through this book, we will help you work smarter, not harder, and with minimum time and maximum results. Because we're mums, we get it!

Kimberley: Diary of a busy mum

Diary entry 1: 'exhaustion'

It's spring 2012 and my typical day looks like this:

- Breastfeed our baby girl.
- Grab a coffee and catch up on the never-ending emails for my husband's new business.
- Feed baby solids.
- Try and rock bub to sleep, because surely she's as exhausted as I am?
- Realise it's already 10am, so bub goes in the bouncer in the bathroom so that I can take a quick shower.
- Have a speedy shower while singing nursery rhymes to keep the peace.
- Get dressed in the first comfortable thing I find.
- Skip breakfast today – no time for nourishment for me.
- Race out the door to try to make it to my scheduled baby-clinic appointment.
- Head home with baby screaming.
- Breastfeed again, still on an empty stomach and my head spinning.
- Quickly eat a piece of cold toast (that will have to be my breakfast and lunch).
- Down another coffee.
- Feed baby lunch.
- Stop baby from repeatedly crawling on top of the TV cabinet.
- Put baby to bed.
- Entertain guests whom I nearly forgot were coming over for afternoon tea.
- Feed baby again when she wakes.
- Race to local shop to scoop up groceries for dinner.
- Breastfeed again.
- Feed baby her dinner.
- Bathe baby.
- Cook dinner.
- Breastfeed baby yet again.
- Welcome husband home, while looking somewhat dishevelled.
- Attempt to put baby to bed, but instead sit in her room rocking her for an hour to get her to sleep, as always.

- Finally I get to eat some dinner.
- I soak in the shower again in an attempt to feel normal.
- Exhausted, I try talk to my husband for ten minutes without yawning, before giving up and heading straight to bed – after all, we both know I'll be awake at least three to six times again tonight.

Not even six months into motherhood and I'm beyond exhausted.

Diary entry 2: 'bone tired'

Our baby girl has reached eleven months of age and suddenly I've started feeling even more tired than usual. I know what it is to have nothing left. I know what people mean by 'bone tired'. I've begun to experience dizzy spells, light-headedness and now nausea. Gulp. Honestly, I didn't think it possible for a human to ever feel this washed out.

Then it dawned on me – this could be morning sickness! Could I be pregnant again? No. I mean, we had talked about it, but surely it was going to take more than a few months to happen? I'm really not sure I'm ready for this. I don't have enough energy to cope *now* – let alone with another miniature human to care for!

I only just finished breastfeeding a few weeks ago and I'm not even sure I've started to feel human again. The pregnancy test is *positive* and within only seconds the result is staring me right in the face: I am pregnant, AGAIN!

Diary entry 3: 'a big change'

I'm too exhausted to write today's diary entry – and with good reason, so I'll keep it short and sweet.

This pregnancy is different from the last. I think that it's got to be a boy, because the morning sickness is just horrid and my body has changed so rapidly. Then we had our scan, which revealed the reason for my extreme morning sickness and overwhelming tiredness. We're having not one, but *two* babies. *Twins*! Someone give me strength! I know I've done this before, but how am I going to do it with two newborns and a 19-month-old? I'm excited but my goodness I'm anxious!

Diary Entry 4: 'life with three'

I have two new darling babies to love and care for. I am the proud mumma of three children and they were all born within 19 months. Like any new mum, I've survived purely on adrenaline for the first few months: I breastfeed two babies at a time while reading a book to my toddler and doing my grocery shopping online. But we've hit the four-month mark now, and that adrenaline has gone. Every ounce of adrenaline has worn off. I have nothing left. I am depleted of energy, health and confidence. My mind feels weak and my body reciprocates the feeling. I've lost the good part of 25kg (4 stone) by breastfeeding and eating on the run all the time, but I feel frail, brain-dead and, worst of all, saggy.

I'm too scared to leave the house on my own with all three kids, but I'm so damn sick of having to rely on other people to help me run my household, and I think I'm actually beginning to go a little stir-crazy. I need to get out. I need – something.

Diary entry 5: 'run mumma, run!'

The twins are five months old – and I feel like I'm a hundred. But I finally cracked it today: I told my husband that I needed to do something otherwise …

I just need to get outside on my own and start exercising again, like I used to. I need to move my body. I used to enjoy running before the kids came along. It was my way of relieving stress. Running used to make me feel good, and so I guess that it's time to start up again.

I went for a run today. It lasted for a grand total of two minutes; this, from a girl who used to run marathons. What has happened to me? I'm not the same person, or at least I don't feel like I am. I want to get the old me back. I want to feel good again.

Diary entry 6: 'a starting point'

A little retrospect. Since my last diary entry, I've tried again and again to run, but everything just felt wrong. My lower back ached, and I didn't have one ounce of core strength. I just felt weak and defeated. It's nothing short of depressing.

But in the depths of my woe-is-me, I had an aha! moment. I decided I had two choices: I could either give up and adopt the attitude of, 'Well, you're a mum now – that's just what happens', or I could explore a different style of training and challenge myself to get some sort of fitness and strength back – emotionally and physically.

The running just wasn't practical or realistic with my busy lifestyle, my kids' needs and my lack of fitness. And so, since then, rather than giving up, I've tried CrossFit, hour-long boot camps with the babies in the stroller, and Pilates. These new fitness regimes worked in a way – and I began to feel better – but the classes were too long and tricky for me to get to. And now I think I've found the solution: I've started doing my own workouts at home. I just thought that anything was better than nothing, so while the kids are eating porridge in their high chairs (smothering it in their hair, over the floor, and now and again getting some in their mouths), I do ten squats. When they are in the bath, I lean against the wall and do some wall push-ups. I'm just a beginner, so doing ten reps is a challenge. Actually, it's hard work. But I know that I have to start somewhere.

Now, I just set myself a goal of around 10 reps for each exercise and aim for two to three rounds (depending on how happy the kids are). Some days I manage to get those rounds in, and on other days I only manage one. I've decided to surrender to the moment and just do what I can, when I can and without putting too much emphasis on feeling guilty if I don't manage what I set out to do. My aim is just to do these workouts twice a week. We'll see how it goes. I'll keep you posted, diary; this is gonna be a challenge!

Diary entry 7: 'building a routine'

I've become addicted to exercising at home. It sounds silly, but it is so much easier for me to get the exercise in when I'm in my own home rather than trying to get us all to a class of some sort. So, what am I doing? Well, I'm just sticking to short-and-sharp exercises, because they clear my mind in an instant, and I can fit them in almost anywhere and at any time. I've found that making this a part of my routine gives me immediate clarity, patience and a degree of serenity. I no longer have to slot in an hour a day to focus on my body. All I need is 15 minutes, and I just do what I can. I am starting to feel alive again. My energy is coming back.

Diary entry 8: 'back in action'

It has been a few months since I started my at-home exercise routine, and everything has changed. I am feeling stronger, dealing with broken sleep better, and I'm so much more relaxed and energised when my husband walks in the door at night. My muscles have even begun to shine through the saggy bits.

It's incredible how just 15-minute bursts of exercise at home make me feel like a different person. I feel more comfortable doing 15 reps now and so I'm adding an extra few rounds to my workouts. I can literally feel myself getting fitter.

When I can, I add an extra workout and I try to aim for three 15-minute sessions a week. I have done a little research too and I've learned about clean eating. This has been my motivation for kick-starting a healthier routine for me and my little family. I've become determined to ensure that our children are fed 'real food' (food that is unprocessed). I'm super-proud of myself for the progress I've made, and I've decided that my kids are certainly not going to survive on a piece of toast all day as I was trying to do not so long ago.

I've discovered that clean eating is about coming back to basics and mostly eating foods that have little to no human intervention. To me, this means foods that you lovingly prepare in your own kitchen and don't just pour from a packet loaded with additives and preservatives so that it can sit on a supermarket shelf for a few years. I've noticed that just by making a few clean-eating changes at home (plus my 15-minute exercises) I have more energy for my kids and more confidence in going out with them. And, as a huge bonus, hubby has even commented on how relaxed I've become. I finally feel like all the pieces are coming together to lay the foundations of a healthy, happy family.

Diary entry 9: 'angel inspiration'

Today I met someone new: Victoria. I was introduced to her through a mutual friend at the local farmers' market and, glancing at her, all I could think was: *Wow*! This girl was like a glowing angel! Her skin was flawless, her hair shiny, her eyes crystal clear and she had a gorgeous figure too. I caught myself wondering if this angel was around my age, but as we got talking, two teenagers came up and stood by her. One of them referred to her as mum. The shock must have registered on my face as I elbowed our mutual friend and not so discreetly asked how old this lady was. When I discovered this radiant girl was in her forties, I nearly flipped.

I think I have found a new-life soul sister. Vicky and I talked over coffee for nearly two hours. We found we could talk for hours on end about health, fitness, family and recipes, and often we even finished each other's sentences (corny, I know). I'm in awe of Vicky's ability to have lived such a healthy lifestyle for nearly two decades – all while raising two gorgeous kids. I think this lady might have just become the final piece of inspiration I need to be the best mum I can be.

Diary entry 10: 'Stay Strong Mummy'

Vicky and I have been catching up every few weeks. She's become my go-to girl for workout ideas, recipes and all the general mum support. It means so much to find someone who understands what it means to be a mum. I've rediscovered the importance of surrounding myself with like-minded people who support me in my efforts to be the best I can be – and we make a great team.

Oh, don't worry, I still have my bad days and testing moments with the kids, but when I share that with Vicky, she simply says, 'It does get easier; just go with it.' Vicky has helped me to remember to breathe a little deeper when things get stressful, and she also reminds me that I'm not alone.

If you read between the lines of my diary, you'll not only see that I live a very busy life as a mum but you'll probably also get an inkling that I'm a crazy, million-mile-an-hour mumma. And for all my craziness, Vicky is my rock. She's the cool, calm and collected one. Vicky is a huge inspiration to me, and I do feel that I am somehow the same for her. She's living proof that following a wholefood diet with short bursts of high-intensity interval training and some strength work is not just a phase, it's a lifestyle. She's been doing it for 20 years.

If Vicky has been a big part of me becoming inspired, fit, healthy and happy, what is it that I do for others? What do I bring to the table? Just as Vicky has inspired me, motivated me and supported me when I needed it most, I do the same for other mums – and I love it.

By sharing my story and supporting other mums in bettering themselves, my business and social media pages took off, and with it, the demands on me suddenly became even greater. It seemed that there were thousands of other mums who shared my journey and who needed motivation and support in feeling better about themselves and their role as a mum. And as I got bombarded with emails and messages from mums all over the world, Vicky would whisper with a smile, 'Just one thing at a time, Kimberley', reminding me again that things are only overwhelming if you allow them to be, and that part of my role on this earth is to inspire others to be and feel great.

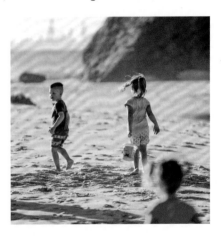

It's now been over three years since I implemented those changes, and it has undoubtedly become a permanent lifestyle for me and my family. I can put my hand on my heart and say, 'I'm feeling fitter, stronger, leaner and healthier than before I had my kids.' And if *I* can do it, so can other mums.

I've shared my diary entries because I'm proud of my journey from independent woman to mother of three children in 19 months. I went from being tired and worn out, feeling overwhelmed, weak and out of my depth, to feeling confident, healthy, energetic and strong. What, then, does this mean for you? Well, I can tell you that regardless of how defeated, isolated, scared or tired you feel right now, motherhood is not a time to lose yourself. It's a time to find your true self so that you can glow with radiance, vitality, fitness and health and be the best role model you can be for yourself and your family. And yes, *you are worth it!*

What's in it for you?

We know how busy you are, so we've got your recipe for success all laid out. No more punishing or exhaustive work, no more costly, unrealistic exercise plans or gym memberships. It's time for you to shine.

With the Stay Strong Mummy Fitness Plan, you'll be on your way to a fitter, healthier and happier you in no time. And we've done all the hard work for you. In this book, you'll find your very own easy-to-achieve fitness plan: it's realistic, time- and cost-effective and fun. And to make things even easier for you, we've got your meals sorted too. What could be better than having your very own fitness and meal plans – all suited to your busy lifestyle as a mum?

How to use this book

You're probably keen to get started, but don't head straight for the recipes or exercises – except for a sneak peak, perhaps. It's important to read through the book to understand how our simple eating and exercise plan works and the benefits you can gain from it. The book is divided into three parts:

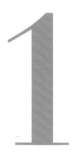

The Mummy Stuff

In Chapter 1 we explain why goal setting is important and how to set sensible goals for yourself that are achievable. You will also find out when is the best time to start on a new fitness regime and how to prepare for it. Chapter 2 explains the importance of being organised and having a routine, as this is the way to ensure you will achieve what you are aiming for in your fitness goals – and also for smoothly functioning family life. We also talk about the importance of sleep and provide some tips for new mums as well as handy hints for mums with twins. We stress the importance of avoiding 'crash and burn' when you basically try to do too much – this tends to mean that your fitness goals end in failure.

In Chapter 3 we help you to stay strong and positive by encouraging you to track your success and your emotions as well as recognising that you need to 'refuel' with love and kindness too – don't be hard on yourself: use our techniques to practise some self-love.

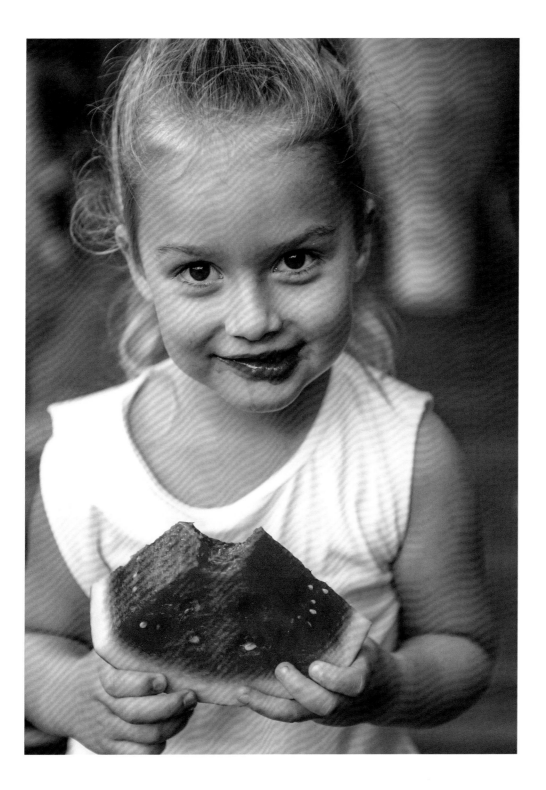

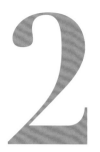

The Yummy Stuff

In Chapter 4 we explain what we mean by 'clean eating', what this involves and how to approach a diet where you avoid processed and pre-prepared convenience foods and instead shop for foods that are in their more natural state. Eating this way will ensure that you and your family are eating the most nourishing meals you can. You will find that when you adopt our clean-eating plan that losing weight becomes much easier. We explain about the main food groups and how it is important to eat these and not to put yourself on highly restrictive diets. In this chapter we also talk about portion sizes – this will be your guide to simple and stress-free weight loss. We also talk you through the foods to buy and those to avoid, and why choosing very good-quality foods is beneficial for our health. Hydration is essential for good health and for weight loss, and in this chapter we explain why. This chapter also sets out your personalised meal plan.

You will find all our recipes in Chapter 5, including some treats for very occasional indulgence. All the recipes are tempting and simple to make and we're sure you'll find them inspiring.

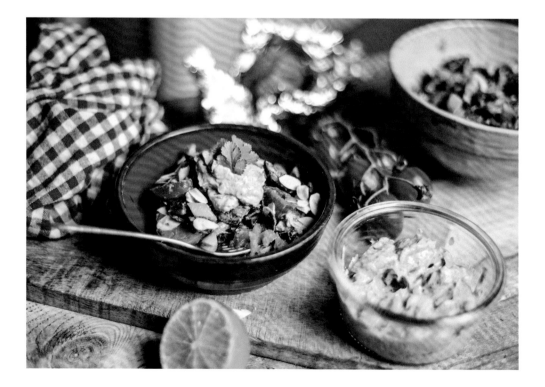

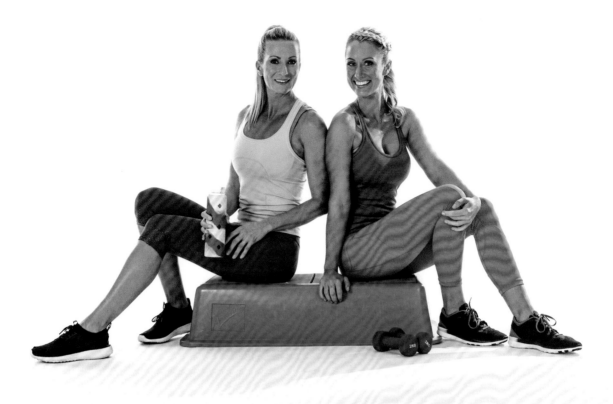

3 **The Strong Stuff** In Chapter 6 we explain how the Stay Strong Mummy Plan is based on a well-tested exercise system that gets the most benefit out of the shortest time frame, ensuring that you will build muscle and burn fat as quickly as possible. In Chapter 7 we set out your Four-Week Fitness Plan, and Chapter 8 contains the exercises themselves plus lots of tips to help you get the most out of them. We also give you hints on how to exercise with your family and how to make it a part of your daily routine with ease.

We want to see you succeed and become the very best mummy you can, so the Stay Strong Mummy Fitness Plan has been tailored just for you. Everything in this book is achievable and, as a complete programme, it will see you kicking your goals with exercise plans of about 15 minutes that can be done in the comfort of your own home, topped with delicious, nutritious, quick-and-easy meals that will help you become slim, trim and feeling just fine. We know you can do it.

Enjoy!

PART I
The **Mummy** Stuff

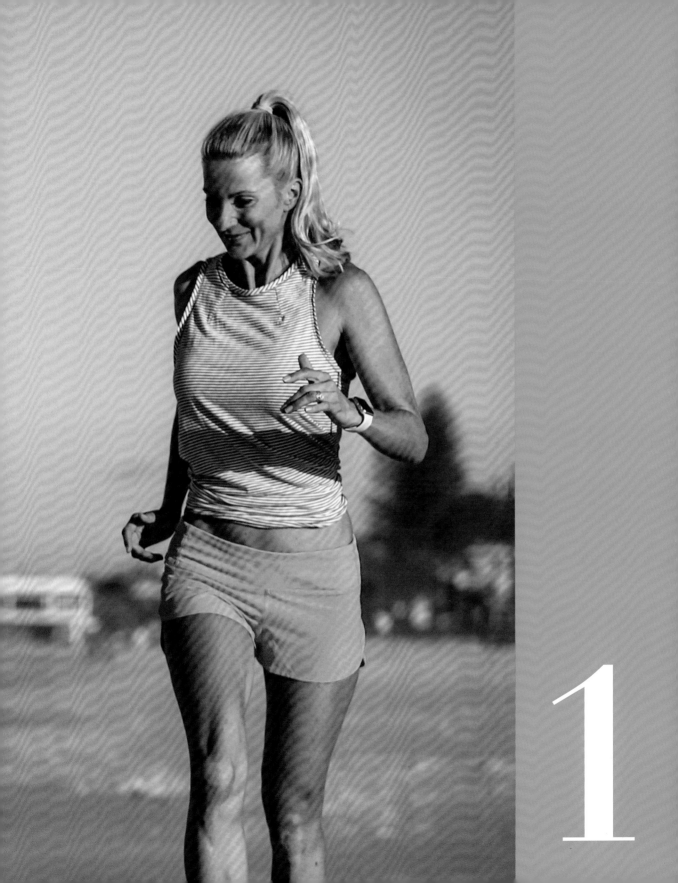

1

CHAPTER 1

Goal Setting for Success

We know your to-do list is already a mile long. And there's a good chance you're reading this with a new baby in your arms, an infant who is asleep or you're racing through these words before you rush out the door to pick up a teenager. However, rather than thinking that you don't have time to set some goals, we want to assure you that the best way to get the results you're after, is to do some planning first. And also to realise that it's not that complicated. We've pared everything down to the basics so that it's as simple as possible for you.

> 'If you want to get somewhere in life and be the best you can be, you have to know where you are going and how you are going to get there!'

Goal setting – why is it important?

We know that we need to capture your attention right here in the first sentence, and already we can hear you thinking: *Goal setting? Really?* Well, bear with us. The truth is that if you want to be as truly awesome as we already know you are, you've got to set some goals. If you want to get somewhere in life and be the best you can be, you have to know where you are going and how you are going to get there. If you can pinpoint what it is you want for yourself and what you want to get from this book, then half the groundwork is already done. And, don't worry, we're here to help with the rest.

Whether you're an avid goal setter already or have never written down a goal in your life, it's important to kick off your Stay Strong Mummy journey by getting old school and having some goals set in action. So grab a pen and paper (*not* your phone or computer) and get ready to *write* down exactly what it is that you want to change in your life. We want you to write down just three goals. Take time to think about what you could choose as your three goals. Without going into too much detail, writing your goals down on paper is crucial, because it reinforces everything your brain is telling your body you want. And, it's nice to write them down in a special journal or in your own diary if you can – somewhere that you can refer back to easily.

To help you get clear on what your three goals could be, we'll be a little more specific. When you write your goals, we want you to break them down into the following: one health goal, one relationship/family goal and one personal (emotional) goal.

It might look something like this:

My goals

1. Increase my fitness and health (lower body-fat levels, tone my body, increase my energy levels).

2. Engage in more quality time with my partner and/or children.

3. Let go of fear, set myself new challenges and use my time more efficiently.

Once you've written down your three goals, it's time to work out how you are going to achieve them and in what time frame; for example:

Strategy and time frame

1. I am going to commit to following the Stay Strong Mummy guide for four weeks.

2. I am going to schedule partner/family time into each day and organise a little family getaway at the end of the month. (Could go camping very inexpensively if budget is tight.)

3. I'm going to work on that new blog, I'm going to learn to meditate, I'm going to spend more time on me, and not feel guilty about it, for one hour each week.

When you are ready to get serious and set goals, it's really important to allow yourself a good hour to sit down to think and write without distraction. The best option might be to allocate time for yourself at night when the kids are in bed. A comfortable space with a cuppa and a candle makes for the perfect goal-setting ambience. Before you write anything, though, just take a few moments to breathe and sit in silence. In silence, we are better able to reflect.

If you're really unsure what your goals should be, just take the time to listen to those inner voices and write down whatever pops up. And if it just doesn't seem to come to you, you can always try this exercise after you've absorbed the wisdom held in the pages you're about to read. Once you have something on paper, you can then formulate it into your goals and keep them in a safe place to refer to once you begin kicking butt. Remember, it's more than fine to change or update your goals as you progress. So are you ready? Let's begin.

Use affirmations

Positive affirmations are powerful reminders that can help turn a negative thought into a positive one. They can instantly change our mindset from negative to positive by reminding us what we have and what to be grateful for. Put positive affirmation quotes on your bathroom mirror and look at them every time you brush your teeth, do your hair or your make-up. It's easier to come across strategically placed affirmations than it is to try to plan them into every day; for example:

I am excited for what today brings

- I am calm and relaxed
- I am happy, I am alive
- I am strong and healthy
- I am enough
- I am supported
- I am beautiful
- I am worthy
- I am confident with my decisions
- I am grateful for all that I have
- I am exactly what my child needs
- I am doing the best I can with what I have

- I am of great worth
- I am patient
- I am not alone; love and support surround me
- I am where I need to be
- I am valued
- I am trusting; this too shall pass
- I am open
- I am strong mentally and physically
- I am excited about today
- I have enough
- I do enough
- I am the source of my own happiness
- I am in a fantastic mood today
- I am joyful every day
- I am organised
- I am fun
- I am proud of myself
- I am in control

When should you start?

We know you're excited and want to start this programme *right now*. That's awesome, but let's take a moment to make sure you're armed with everything you need so that you're ready to rock. Here are our top tips to get you off to a strong start with the Stay Strong Mummy Plan.

'Let's take a moment to make sure you're armed with everything you need so that you're ready to rock!'

- There is something so sparkly and energising about a new week, and so we recommend kicking off this programme on a Monday: new week, new start, new enthusiasm, new *you*.

- Spend some time at the weekend visiting a farmers' market or getting your grocery shopping done for the week. (Remember to write out your food list for the week and take it with you.)

- Make sure you have written your goals down and put them in a safe place.

- Place some positive affirmation cards on your bathroom mirror so that you can look at them while brushing your teeth every day.

- Tell your family and friends that you're embarking on this exciting new challenge and will be making some changes. Let them know how important their support will be to your success. Be aware of anyone who immediately says, 'That sounds so hard' or 'Why would you want you to do that?' or 'How will you have time?' Negative comments and negative people make for a more difficult journey to success.

- Choose your company wisely over the next month – it pays to be around positive and motivated people. And, *yes* – you do have a choice as to whom you surround yourself with.

- Make yourself accountable. Have you got another mummy friend who could do this programme with you? It really does help to find a Stay Strong Mummy buddy who can talk it through with you once every few days. If not, head over to StayStrongMummy.com.

- Detox your pantry and fridge – get rid of all the processed and packaged foods (more about that in Chapter 4).

- Make yourself some sweet but healthy treats and have them stored away for when cravings arise. You will find a few in the recipe section in Chapter 5.

- Have your first week of workouts (as explained in Chapter 7) planned out and written down in a training diary. It helps to map your progress if you write down your feelings after each workout.

You're only one workout away from a good mood

- Whenever a negative thought pops up during a workout, become aware of it and push it to the side. Don't give in because you think you *can't* do it. We're here to break through that negative self-talk once and for all.

- Whenever you find yourself looking at excess skin, muffin tops, stretch marks, and so on, take a deep breath, smile and think how lucky you are to have your children – and get straight back into it.

- Go to bed early. Turn the phone off, limit or eliminate distractions and turn the TV off. This is *your* time now.

- Get in that beauty sleep and get ready to transform your life!

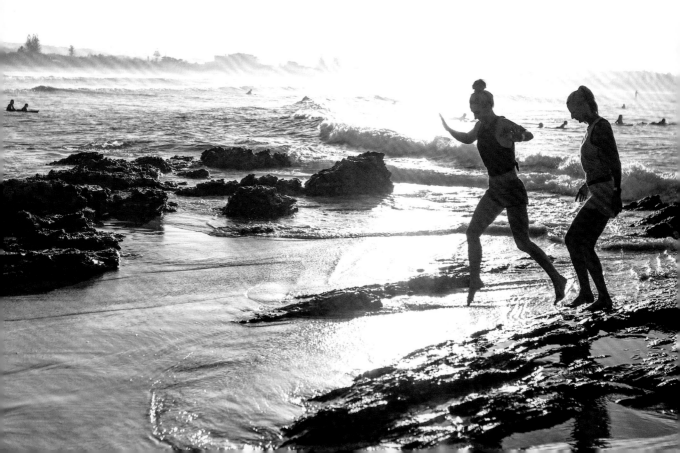

CHAPTER 2

Routine and Organisation are Essential

Many mums like to get back into some sort of fitness regime soon after having a baby. Whether it's the challenge of moving your body again without a hefty weight sitting on your pelvis or an outlet to shake off any stress and tension, or maybe to strengthen, tone and lose that additional baby weight, it's a wonderful and admirable trait to want to get back into exercise after becoming a mum. But (here comes the 'but' again), if there is one thing that we have learnt from our own motherhood journeys, it's to ensure that you don't rush the process. We want you to make lifestyle changes once and for all. And the best way to do that, particularly if you have a new baby, is to ensure that you are prepared and that you take a balanced approach to your health and fitness.

Avoid the crash and burn

A lot of women start out on a new diet and exercise plan filled with motivation and inspiration only to find that they crash and burn within a week. There are many factors that can come into play when it comes to giving up on exercise, but mainly it's because it's simply not a maintainable programme for them and their lifestyle. Those women who give up are likely to be overworking or setting unrealistic goals when it comes to health and fitness.

Some of the contributing factors of giving up when you're just starting out with a healthy life overhaul could include: (a) working out six days a week for an hour at a time; (b) restricting major food groups and calories, and (c) simply becoming utterly exhausted each and every day. If you don't make a planned fitness session or manage to prepare that healthy meal, your disappointment levels will go through the roof and you'll be left feeling like a failure. And that is precisely why so many people take an all-or-nothing approach to health and fitness: it's either all systems go, or it's completely switched off and time to binge-eat on the couch.

You need to be especially careful as a mother, because you're often lacking sleep, and your exercise regime needs to be energising you rather than depleting you. Our programme has been designed to nourish and not punish you at a time when you need support, not guilt.

Although at times making changes to your diet, fitness and lifestyle might feel a little challenging, rest assured that you'll be bouncing around with an abundance of energy and new-found strength once you get going. And you won't be alone; one of the greatest things we have learnt as busy mothers is to surrender to the moments. Realise that some days will work effortlessly and you'll get that workout in and nourish yourself as you should, and other days, when you've got an unsettled newborn, a teething toddler or you are at the beck and call of an older child, you may end up missing that workout. Rather than let the negative chitter-chatter enter into your head, just remind yourself that tomorrow is a new day. Get up earlier the next day, stay up a little later in the evening, find a window of opportunity and just go with it. When you've got some routine and structure to your days, it's not as hard to pencil in a session. The key is to not let that one day spiral into a week or two of no activity, but to get back into the swing of things as soon as you can.

Build in some structure to your day

As mums, we know just how much some routine and structure helped us to run a healthy, happy and most-of-the-time calm household. Those first few months are often chaotic and an exhaustive blur; a never-ending production line of feeding, trying to get babies to sleep, playing with older kids and doing chores.

We know that your washing line is full to the brim every single day, and we know that you sometimes wake anything up to eight times a night to tend to all the kids at some stage. We know that you're exhausted, and we know what it feels like to have everyone want a piece of you – to the point where the only communication you have with your husband is a quick nod as you pass each other in the hallway at 2am as you go from room to room.

By six months, however, if you haven't already, it's time to focus on adding some structure and routine to your days, and when you do you'll become more aware of the little wave of calmness entering the household. Not a huge wave, just a little one – but it will be enough to make the days flow a lot easier.

Once you implement routine and structure for the basics of parenting, you'll find that you can do it with healthy eating and exercise as well. The result will be a much happier, more relaxed and more energetic family unit. You'll still have hectic days where absolutely nothing goes to plan. And you'll probably still be in your pyjamas when your partner gets home some evenings, but the bulk of the days will begin to feel a lot smoother having that bit of structure and routine. The same can be said when you apply routine and structure to your eating and exercise habits.

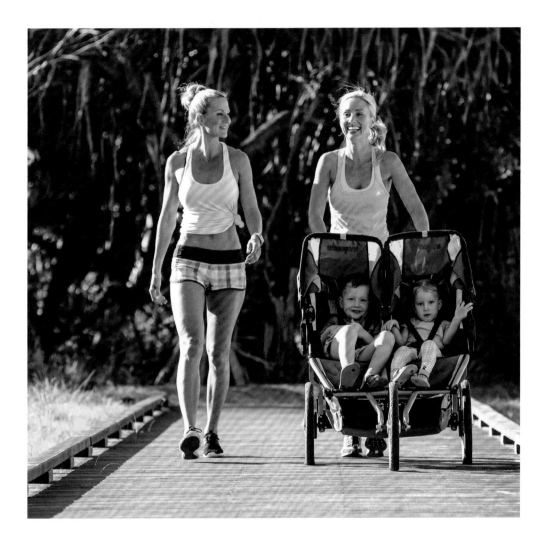

Routine and structure do require some organisation. It's the little things that make a big difference when it comes to organisation, whether it's setting up for bath time, cooking dinner in the morning, making breakfast for the following day, packing the car the night before a daycare or school drop off, setting up play areas outside for a mummy/ playtime workout that afternoon or laying out the kids' clothes the evening before. We love being a few steps ahead of our little tribes (most of the time) because we know the benefits first hand. One really valuable question to ask yourself is, 'What can I do today that will help take the pressure off tomorrow?' This question alone is a great way to begin the journey of getting organised.

Babies and routine

How many times have you googled: 'how do you get a baby to sleep?' in those early months of being a first-time mum? If you parented for the first time before Google became the go-to reference point, there's a good chance you found your overtired eyes transfixed on numerous parenting books in search of the answers to the very same question.

There are millions of different industry experts, books, websites and apps out there, all telling mums something different with regard to sleep advice, and rightly so. Every single baby and mother is different, so of course there are always going to be countless different ways to get a baby to sleep. It is one of the hottest questions for new mums, as sleep deprivation can be extremely stressful and draining for a lot of us.

'We wanted to include this section because when we were first-time mums it's probably the first section we would flick to in the depths of our sleep-deprived days and nights with little babies'

Our most important piece of advice for new mummies out there who are dealing with broken sleep is to know that it will pass. You will get eight hours of sleep again, one day soon. It's really hard to see that light at the end of the tunnel when you're in the thick of it, but it will shine through eventually.

Spending time on your health and fitness is actually a wonderful way to combat the broken sleep of motherhood. Clean foods and exercise will help your body build energy! The key is to focus on nourishing, and not punishing, yourself (our plan is built on this foundation.)

The wonderful thing about the online world is that experiences, information and research is available to anyone, anywhere and at any time. If you're looking for help in getting your baby to sleep, then explore different techniques, network with other like-minded mums and find some tactics that you feel comfortable with on your own parenting journey. Whatever it is you choose to do, have confidence in your ability. You are the most equipped and experienced person on this earth to parent your baby. Don't ever doubt it. Sure, talk to other women, read up on different experiences and get amongst a mothers' group for on-going support, but always remind yourself that you are enough – trust your instinct.

Here are some tips that helped us:

- Create a warm, loving and nurturing sleep environment for your baby. For the first few months you might find it easier to have them close by or next to you, so that you can simply reach over and pick them up to feed.

- Ensure your baby's room is dark and at a comfortable temperature. Keep in mind that 4am is often the coolest part of the night (and a common time for babies to wake!).

- Give your baby a comforter of your choosing. It could be a little blanky, bunny, a fluffy piece of material – whatever works for you. You can try putting the comforter down your top when your baby isn't in bed so that it picks up your scent. Babies love smelling their mother and it's often calming for them to be given the comforter at sleep time.

- Get a midwife, child health nurse or health visitor to show you how to swaddle your baby tightly and correctly. Their arms and legs can distract them and wake them if they flinch and move their limbs suddenly. Babies love being snug (just like in your tummy), so swaddling can help to keep everything firmly in place and keep baby feeling secure.

- It can often help to relax babies and induce sleep if you put on soft 'white noise' or relaxing music at sleep time. Whatever you choose, it can be helpful to use the same sound each time they rest. With repetition and routine, your baby will come to recognise sleep time and will also be less likely to wake to other noises.

- Learn about babies' sleep cycles and the different modes of sleep (light sleep and deep sleep). It's all very fascinating and informative. There's a difference between a sleep and nap!

- Putting your baby to sleep at the time each day can help set their body clock, just like ours. It does mean that you spend a lot of time at home in those first few months, but it does really help them settle and get into a good sleeping routine.

- If you have a baby monitor in your baby's room, it pays to cover the red light on the camera, as it can be distracting for them.

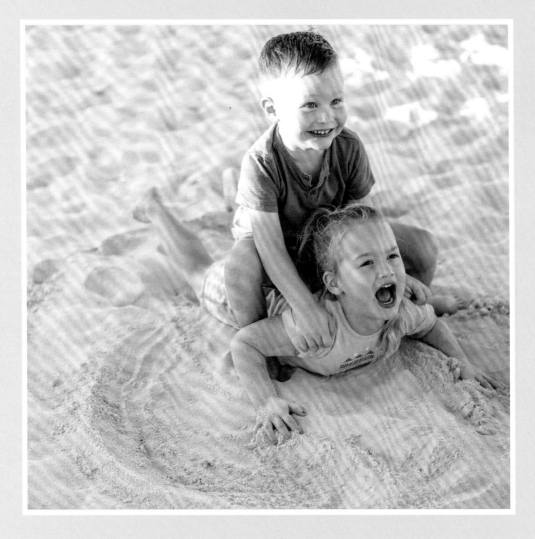

- Always make sure your baby is well-fed, burped and has a clean nappy before sleep time. Some days we would try and pat and stroke our babies to sleep and sit on the floor beside their cots (some days for hours on end!); other days we would rock or feed them. If we did rock or feed them, we would generally try to put them in their own bed just prior to them drifting off. It helps to teach them that they are safe, secure and able to drift off on their own accord.

- Kids learn best from praise and positive reinforcement. When your baby begins to catch on to the whole sleeping thing, each time they wake (except when it's in the middle of the night), you should make a fuss about congratulating them on sleeping well. Once they are fully awake, open up the curtains or turn the light on and let them know that it is 'awake' and 'playtime' now.

- To help your little one wind down at night, a regular, calm night-time routine can be great. Where possible, aim to bath or shower your baby at the same time each night. After the bath, try to keep them in their own room, with the lights dim, white noise on and read, softly sing or give them a gentle massage. Let them know it's time for quiet and peaceful rest.

- Doing milk feeds in your baby's room, rather than in front of a bright and loud TV can also help them relax. This is tricky when you have siblings charging down the hallway or yelling out 'what's for dinner, mummy?', but maybe they might like to join in on the quiet time, or you could try setting up some little snacks or quiet activities for them while you tend to baby. Remember, this isn't forever – it's just in the early stages.

- Everyone parents differently and each and every child is different. We encourage you to do your own research on the latest Government, child safety and sudden-infant-death (SID) guidelines to ensure you are meeting the safety requirements, and, of course, do what works for you and your family.

Extra help for mums of twins

If you're a new mother of multiples, having a gentle routine and some structure to your days is even more likely to help create harmony in your home. When you've got two babies (or more) to care for, then you need to be as organised as possible. If you breastfeed, there's a good possibility that you'll be sitting on the couch for up to two

Tip: Persistance is important

Our babies thrived on a gentle routine. We found that they loved to know what was coming next and felt safe and secure. When we started putting them to bed at the same time each day, had their feeds at roughly the same times and play times at similar times, they eventually began to enjoy their sleep time more. When they finally got that sleeping thing sorted, they enjoyed their awake times more too, fed a lot better and were more happy and relaxed.

'As a mum, you'll learn to use your time wisely. As a mum of multiples, this is even more crucial'

hours or longer at a time. And then there's the burping, topping them up and changing nappies. When they're really young, you'll probably just get through this and it will feel like it's time to start over again.

As a mum, you'll learn to use your time wisely. As a mum of multiples, this is even more crucial. We know that being a mum means you're busy all day. Aside from the feeding, you're likely to hardly sit down all day – but you probably wouldn't have it any other way.

- We know how exhausted you are when the sun comes up each day, but if you can set an alarm and muster the energy to wake about half an hour before your babies do, it will mean that you probably get in a shower and cup of tea (or one of our amazing smoothies, see pages 89–90) before your baby duties begin. Even if you can't manage this every morning, when you do you'll feel so much more refreshed and able to cope with what the day brings.

- If you can, go into feeds prepared and have everything you'll need: breastfeeding pillows, bouncers at your feet, snacks and toys for the other children, bibs, water, nappies and wipes all in the one place and in reach – it will make everything seem that little bit easier and less stressful.

- When settling your twins to sleep, try having their cots 1m apart from each other so that you can sit on the floor between them with one arm in each cot patting them both in sync. This saves you time and energy, and it gets both babies into the same routine – after all, there is only one of you.

- Invest in a good double pram that you can easily manage when you go for walks and outings.

- Try to get outside at least once a day, even if it's just for a five-minute walk in the fresh air. If you can get out, you'll always feel a little more energised when you return.

- In the early days, it is important for you to rest when your babies are having a daytime nap. But once you start to find your flow, those precious hours during the day when they are asleep can be a great time for you to 'get ahead' with personal stuff. It's a great time to cook dinner, enjoy a workout and spend some time on your goals or passions. It's also a great time to set up for the afternoon 'rush hour', i.e. get everything ready for bath time, set the dinner table, set up highchairs or feeding stations and so on.

- Go into bath time prepared. Get absolutely everything out that you'll need. If you've got other children, let them be the bath time 'boss'. Get them to feel part of the process and tell you what to do. If you've had a big day and your babies are unsettled,

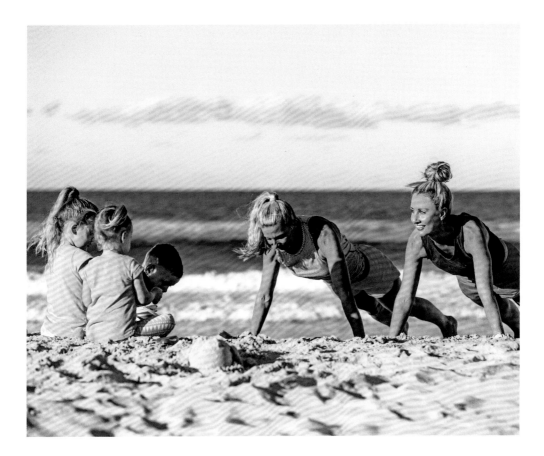

just bathe one baby on alternate days (yes, it's okay). This way your babies will bathe every second day and you can just lightly sponge them down on alternate days. Now and again it is okay if a newborn only bathes every second day.

- Take time for yourself whenever you can. Enjoy the workouts we've set out in this book – they may just become your sanity check. You need two super-strong arms with multiple babies and, as they grow, they will both still want you at the same time and you'll love being strong enough to pick them both up.

- When it all gets too much ensure your babies are well fed and have clean nappies, then take off for a quiet drive. Put some relaxing music on in the car, make yourself a protein smoothie and hit the road. Whenever you need a little time out, your car can provide just that.

Mummy Mantra

I am where I need to be

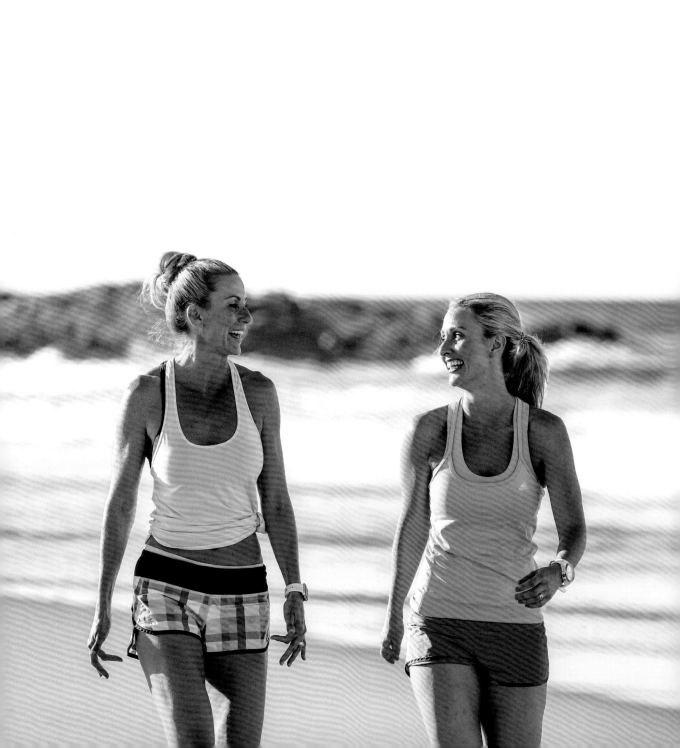

CHAPTER 3

How to Stay Strong and Positive

Our programme is a four-week fitness and health plan but it has been designed to empower and educate you to make life-long changes. Once the initial four weeks is over, you may choose to repeat the plan if you feel you need continued guidance. Alternatively, you may feel ready to embark on this new way of life on your own and simply use this book as a reference, and the programme as a framework for your lifestyle, for many years to come. It should also serve as a valuable emotional 'companion'. Refer back to it for reminders on tracking your success and staying focused on the positive powers of a healthy mindset.

'It often takes commitment before the motivation starts to flow. Make the commitment and have the discipline to follow through with your plan'

Track your success

When your goals have been set and you are ready to start the Stay Strong Mummy Fitness Plan, we recommend a few different ways to track your progress. They will help you to stay on track and give you that little push of extra motivation each week.

Keep in mind that improving your health and losing stubborn body fat can take time, so it's important to be patient. This book and programme have been written for you to make life-long changes, not just for the four weeks of the programme. Some people may find that they lose weight within the first week, others might not budge until week three and others might only just start to see the light by week four. Everyone is different and you need to acknowledge that before you start.

Emotional tracking

In addition to tracking measurements, a big part of your progress is to track your emotional state as well. They both work hand in hand. Over this four-week period, in addition to the fitness and food, we want you to work on letting go of any negative self-talk, we want you to deal with any emotional baggage you're holding on to, and we want you to let go of all that stuff and clutter that is taking up space in your head. When you deal with the emotional stuff, you'll notice the physical results get better and better too. A big part of our tracking is *how you feel*. Have a special diary (yep, go back to your teenage years and get yourself a new diary that no one else can read) and each week document how you feel. It can be one sentence, or it could be five pages long. But every Monday, write in your diary. Check in with yourself: 'How are my energy levels, my moods and anxiety levels?', 'What things am I constantly thinking about?', 'What am I going to make a conscious effort to do this week to stop the negative chitter-chatter going on in my head?' How you feel is a very important indicator of your progress.

Fat-loss tracking

Try not to get too obsessed with what the bathroom scales are telling you. It wouldn't matter if we were to say to you, 'Don't jump on the scales', because the reality is that most of you will do that – and the numbers on there *do* matter when you're starting out. If you do wish to use the scales, just keep in mind that it's important not to get fixated on them. Remember, we are aiming for life-long changes. When you are only concerned about the numbers on a scale and seeing that as a way to make or break your day, it's not a healthy mindset. Having your period, holding onto excess fluid, not releasing your bowels, and the time of day can all give inaccurate results on the scales. Plus, we want to lose body fat and increase muscle mass. Muscle weighs more than fat – fact.

We recommend tracking your physical (fat loss) results using these three easy options:

1 **Take before-and-after photos.** No one needs to see these. They can be taken using your phone's self-timer camera or you can ask someone close to you to take them for you. Take a photo first thing in the morning (before breakfast) in the same spot, wearing the same underwear, using the same camera. Take it on the first day you start this programme and on the last day. Our dream is for you to continue this programme well after four weeks. You can choose to repeat it, or you might feel armed with knowledge and motivation to keep going on your own. We recommend that every month you take that same progress photo.

2 **Take your waist measurement.** This needs to be taken on the days you start weeks 2 and 4. Simply wrap a tape measure around your waist using your belly button as a start and finishing point. Dropping size in this area is a good indication that you are losing body fat.

3 **Be patient.** Stress and lack of sleep can stall fat loss. This is due to the stress hormone cortisol. We know as mums that eight hours' sleep isn't always possible, but start to use your downtime more wisely. Rather than sitting with your phone when you've got 15 minutes to yourself, try downloading a meditation app. A lot of yogis believe that 15 minutes of deep meditation is equivalent to 3–4 hours' sleep.

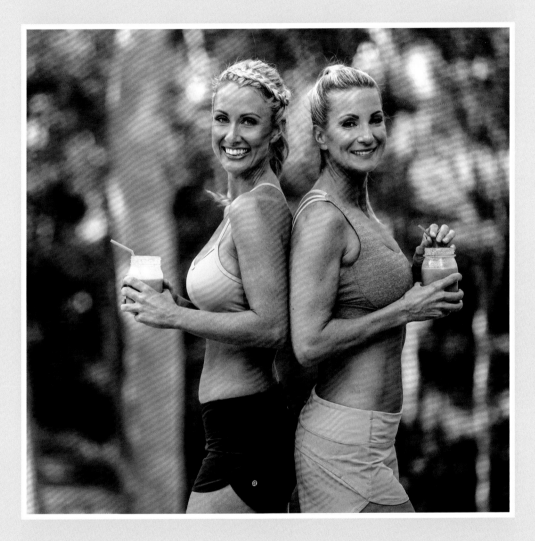

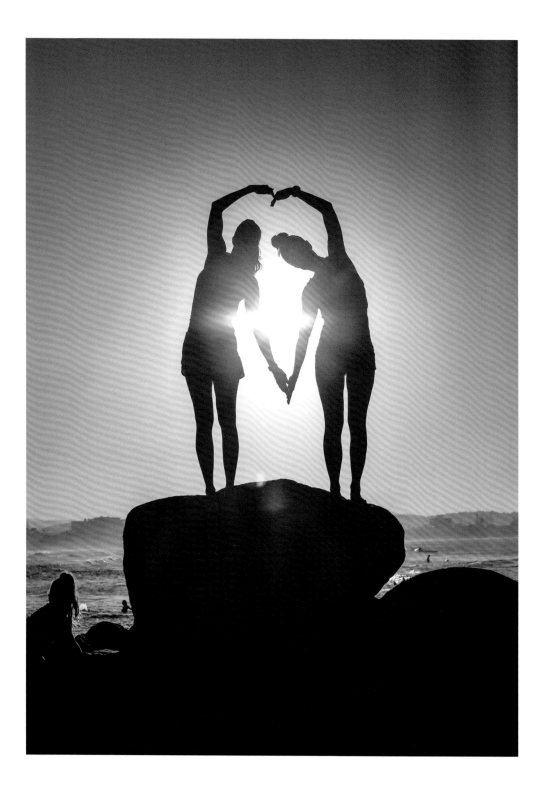

Aim for positivity

A positive mindset is one of the most powerful tools we can harness. And, it's also one of the hardest things for people to maintain in this day and age. We wanted to include this section so you can refer back to it on those more challenging days and remind yourself that learning to look for the good in every situation is contagious once you start changing your mindset.

- It often takes commitment before the motivation starts to flow. Make the commitment and have the discipline to follow through with your plan.
- It takes 21 days to form a new habit, so commit to making changes for four weeks and you'll find the motivation naturally kicks in.
- On the tough days when you're sleep deprived or have a sick baby, or when you just can't seem to get into the swing of things, focus on food rather than exercise. Rest on the couch with your loved ones (while having a smoothie, for example) or head off to the shops to stock up on groceries, cook yourself an extra-special lunch, then focus on nourishing yourself and your family.
- You can let the day run you, or you can run the day.
- If you feel yourself slipping, jump online and start talking to other mums in your mothers' groups or via social media. Inspiration can be found within minutes of talking and connecting with like-minded mums.

'When you are only concerned about the numbers on a scale and seeing that as a way to make or break your day, it's not a healthy mindset'

Self-love for mums

Being a mother is one of the most blessed and greatest gifts we will ever receive. No matter where, when, how or why a baby comes into your arms, when you're given the opportunity to be a mum, a whole new part of your heart opens up in a way like never before. In addition to such joy that motherhood brings you, at times it can also be extremely challenging and tiring. It can push you to your limits, test your patience and take you on a rollercoaster ride that feels like it is only allowed to stop for short moments at a time.

But we're here to tell you that, as mothers, it is so important to jump off that rollercoaster and slow down now and again. You're expending a great deal of energy, day in and day out, caring for your little people around the clock, and if you don't pull back and spend some time refuelling emotionally and physically, you'll come to a screaming halt.

Refuel your mind with acts of self-love and refuel your emotions by spending time on your relationships, goals, passions and just taking the time to 'check in' with yourself now and again. All of these things make such a difference to your energy levels, clarity of mind, health, fitness and happiness. There is a wide range of techniques you can use to refuel your emotions, so there is certain to be one or two that you might like to try.

Self-love techniques

The art of self-love will mean different things to different people but essentially it comes down to creating a space in your schedule to quiet your mind or taking 'time out' to do something that will calm and invigorate you.

- Download a meditation clip of your choice and aim to listen to it for a few minutes at least once a week (once a day is great), either early in the morning or last thing at night.

- If you're struggling with meditation or spending some quiet time with yourself, head off to a local yoga class for some guidance. A yoga class only needs to be once a week to have tremendous benefits. You can also practise some of the poses at home; that'll also help.

- Surround yourself with positive affirmations at home. (See the 'mummy mantras' in this book for ideas. As we saw in Chapter 1, affirmations are great for sticking on the fridge, your desk or on the bathroom mirror.)

> ' Refuel your mind with acts of self-love, and refuel your emotions by spending time on your relationships, goals, passions and just taking the time to check in with yourself now and again '

- Spend time working on your own goals, interests and passions. They are often the things that you think about a lot of the time, or spend your time researching and reading about. Whether it's art, reading, cooking, studying, fashion or blogging, and so on, make a little time to allow your attention to flow there.

- Let go of past hurts, mistakes and grudges. Although this is not always easy, choosing to forgive will free up more energy for yourself and the ones you love.

- Put your phone away, close the laptop, turn off the TV and walk outside to feel the sun on your face or to look at the stars. Take deep breaths and feel a connection to your surroundings.

- Stop comparing yourself to others – and make a list of your strengths. Write down the things you know you are good at. Think about the skills you used before you had kids and how you can incorporate them into your life now.

- This is an oldie but a goodie! Run yourself a warm bath, dim the lights, light a candle, grab a book or play some relaxing music. Immerse yourself in bubbles and relax.

- Sometimes just sitting in front of the TV and doing your nails with a candle burning is enough to help you switch off.

- Go for a walk and listen to your mind. Make a conscious effort to pull yourself up every time a negative thought pops up, and replace it with a positive one.

- Look at yourself in the mirror every day for a week and say to yourself, 'I am beautiful inside and out.' And believe it.

- If you have young children and find yourself having to feed overnight, practise closing your eyes and meditating at the same time. Four o'clock in the morning is believed to be one of the most spiritual times of the day, according to yogis. And 15 minutes of meditation is equivalent to about 3 hours of deep sleep.

Helpful app timers for busy mums

In Part 3 we'll be explaining all about how our exercise plan works. Your aim will be for short bursts of intense activity – called HIIT – and this ensures that you will get the most out of your exercise time and really get the fat burning and the muscle toned.

High-intensity interval training (HIIT) is exactly that: *intense*! And the last thing you want to be focusing on is how many reps you have done or how long you have to go during a workout. You want to get in there and get the job done with *total focus*! This is why we prefer to work out to an interval timer app. It does all the work for you so that you can focus 100 per cent on the exercise you are performing at the time.

These apps are a fantastic tool for busy mums to get organised and stay motivated. Plan your workout and set your timer the night before. You simply set the timer to the recommended work and rest period for each workout by programming in the number of exercises and the number of total rounds. Your timer will prompt you when to work and when to rest and advise you of how many rounds you have left. It's almost like you have set an appointment with your own personal trainer.

There is a variety of different interval timers that you can buy online very inexpensively. They all do a similar job. Check them out – you might just save yourself time and energy.

Mummy Mantra

You can let the day run you, or you can run the day

PART 2
The Yummy Stuff

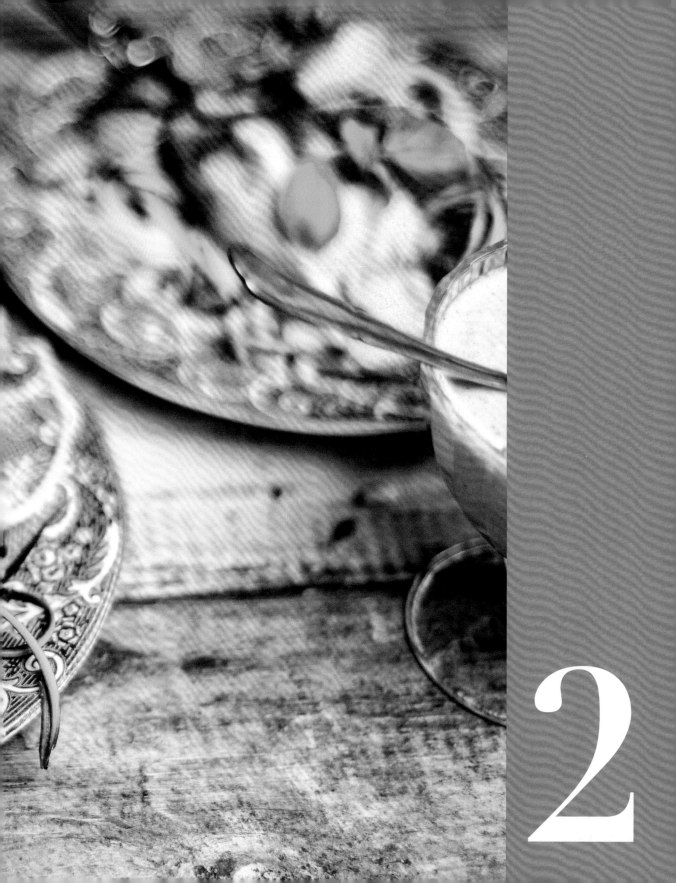

2

CHAPTER 4

You Can Benefit from Whole Foods and Clean Eating

You've probably heard people say they're on a 'clean-eating diet', but what exactly does this mean? It's simple. Clean eating is all about choosing foods that have no added chemicals, artificial flavourings or preservatives to alter the taste or enhance shelf life.

Eating clean, healthy, whole foods every day is a conscious choice that takes practice, but it can vastly improve the quality of your life, health, fitness and state of mind. When choosing clean foods for you and your family, think of quality over quantity.

'Getting back to basics and back to whole foods doesn't have to be time-consuming'

Why is clean eating important?

Generally, people who eat clean do so because they want to nourish their body with foods that are as natural and nutrient-rich as possible. A dedicated whole-food eater becomes more aware of what has gone into the food that goes into their mouth to nourish their bodies. Clean eating means eating foods that are as close to their natural state as possible. These are whole foods and they include fresh vegetables, fruit, meat, fish, poultry, eggs, nuts and seeds. Organic foods are obviously the best choices if you can afford them, but just eating foods that have not been previously prepared is excellent too.

Although it sounds as if it might take a lot of effort, as with any diet you'll always have options to ease your way into learning about and immersing yourself into clean-eating habits. With the right information and support, clean eating does not have to be costly or time-consuming, nor does it have to mean lifestyle upheaval.

Although most of us might easily be able to imagine how much damage processed food does to our insides, for many of us buying natural foods is not necessarily a first choice when it comes to regular eating habits. Clean eating doesn't have to mean changing all the meals you eat, however, nor does it mean you have to miss out. It's actually about making healthy choices and making it a way of life, rather than simply following a diet.

At first, it might take a little extra time to get to know the products to buy and what constitutes whole food, but once you're familiar with the right products it's easy to maintain a clean-eating way of life and, what's more, it can be very rewarding.

Clean eating is a main component of the Stay Strong Mummy Plan for several reasons. The foods that you eat affect your mind, body and soul. Clean foods are real foods that are full of nutrients and life, and they vibrate through every cell of your being, leaving you feeling refreshed, full of energy and boasting an increased clarity of mind. Your diet is not only related to your physical self, it's also related to your feelings, thoughts and emotions.

Fuelling your body with clean whole foods every day will give you vitality, strength and clarity. Whole foods promote happiness in your life, while helping you to maintain a healthy lifestyle and weight. We really do believe that clean eating prolongs life. It truly is nature's best preventative and natural medicine, and it will help to keep you feeling and looking young and vibrant. Getting back to basics and returning to using whole foods is essential for good health and it doesn't have to take hours to prepare – simply being organised is the key.

What are whole foods?

Whole foods are those that have received very little or no intervention by humans. They have not been processed or tampered with. They are foods that have come from nature rather than the result of a factory or industrial process.

Remember the kinds of foods that our grandparents always ate? Vegetables were picked from the garden or bought from the greengrocer or market, milk and eggs came from the dairy, a local shop or farmer, and meats from animals that had been grazing on grass came directly from the butcher. These types of foods were lovingly prepared over a hot stove and they didn't require added artificial flavours or colouring. These are whole foods.

Your guide to whole foods

If you avoid anything that needs an ingredient label, you will be sure to be buying whole foods. Here are the foods to choose:

- Fresh fruit and vegetables – aim for locally sourced, in season and organic where possible.
- Grains – look for 100 per cent whole grains. For flours, look for minimal processing, non GMO (genetically modified), and do not buy 'enriched' or bleached flour.
- Dairy products (milk, yogurt, cheese) and eggs – choose organic, unsweetened and pasture-raised where possible. Note that today many dairy cows do not graze in fields but are raised in barns. Barn-raised cattle will be fed some grass, but they are also

fed grains. Milk and dairy products from cows that graze in the fields is preferable. Similarly, eggs often come from hens raised in tightly packed barns, which adversely affects the hens' quality of life. Frequently they have to be fed antibiotics. Eggs from free-range hens are preferable. We talk more about produce from free-range and grass-fed animals on page 68.

- Meat (beef, lamb and pork), poultry and fish – choose pasture-fed beef and lamb, free-range pork and poultry, and wild-caught fish.

There will be times when you have to buy foods that are packaged or canned. In these cases, try to buy as basic foods as possible. Avoid the following ingredients and additives too:

- Artificial flavours.
- Enriched wheat, corn (unless organic).
- Hydrogenated oils such as palm, kernel, soya bean, corn oil, rapeseed oil.
- MSG (monosodium glutamate), artificial colourings, potassium benzoate and sodium benzoate, sodium chloride.
- Sugar, high-fructose corn syrup, artificial sweeteners such as sucralose, aspartame, NutraSweet and Equal, Xylitol, Sorbitol, saccharin, Splenda.
- Soya (unless organic or fermented), soy lecithin.

The truth about soya/soy products

Once known as a 'healthy' food, soya and soy products have gained a bad rap over the years after extensive research. A number of studies have shown that some soya products can block absorption of major nutrients, such as calcium, magnesium, iron and protein, and can cause swelling of the pancreas, inhibiting regular thyroid function and disrupting the endocrine system. Soy phytoestrogens also have the potential to cause infertility and to promote breast cancer.

However, it's important to note that some soya products are acceptable. These are organic fermented tempeh, miso and tamari sauce, as they have not been cross-contaminated with other soy products.

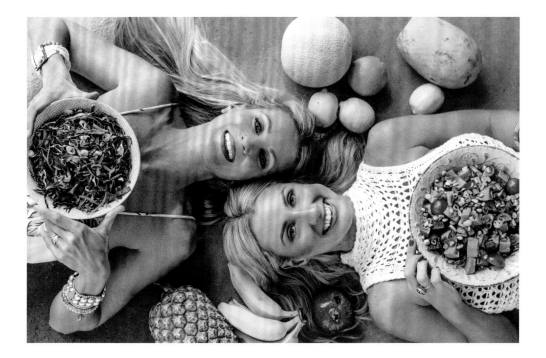

How are foods and emotions linked?

You've heard it before – and it's *true*: we actually *are* what we eat! When you become a conscious eater, you will soon realise that food affects you on an emotional level just as much as it does on a physical one. Have you ever noticed the difference in how you feel when you start the day with a nutritious breakfast (such as a veggie-loaded omelette or a super-green protein smoothie – you'll find both in our recipe section) compared with how you feel if you skip breakfast or grab something that has little or no nutritional value, such as white toast with jam or some sugary low-fat cereal? When you start the day nourishing your body, you are setting up your day for success – rather than failure. Your concentration, productivity and mood will depend on how you fuel your body. Good, wholesome food will give you an increased feeling of control, energy and well-being.

When you fuel your body with unhealthy additives and foods, such as sugar, highly processed breads and junk food, your body has to work harder to process it. This extra work leaves you feeling heavy, tired, depleted, depressed and, strangely enough, even though you're full, craving more food. This type of eating is like being on a never-ending rollercoaster ride: you are up, then down, up, then down, and you eat more to get up again quickly only to end up more tired, anxious and hungry. It's a vicious circle.

Cravings – what your body is really telling you

Contrary to popular belief, cravings are not a sign of weakness. Your body is a very smart, complex tool that is communicating with you every second of the day. When you experience cravings for particular foods, it's your body's way of trying to tell you something – so listen. A craving generally means that your body is out of balance and that you are not absorbing or obtaining the nutrients you need from the food you are eating. It's an alarm bell of sorts that you need to make changes to your diet, food intake or lifestyle.

So how do we interpret what our body is trying to tell us and make changes for the better? Don't worry, we've got your back, and we know just how to interpret those body messages.

Here's a list of some of the most common alarm bells that your body will give you when you need to make changes to the foods and nutrients you're taking in.

Your cravings decoded

Chocolate – your body needs avocados, whole grains, dark leafy greens, and, dare I say, dark chocolate (70% cocoa or higher).

Sugary foods – your body doesn't really want sugar, it actually needs nuts, chicken, fresh fruit, beef, oily fish, eggs, dairy, veggies or whole grains.

Bread, pasta, carbs – your body needs protein. Time to get a dish of high-protein foods: meat, oily fish, nuts, beans or chia seeds.

Fatty foods – what do you like best? Organic milk, nut milk and green leafy vegetables are all good sources.

Salty foods – your body would rather have nuts and seeds than a dose of salt.

Also note these important factors

Dehydration – when you are dehydrated there is a good chance you are going to crave food. Drink a big glass of water before you reach for food.

Sleep deprivation – this plays a part in cravings. When you're a new mum there is a good chance you are going to be sleep-deprived, and if you don't get enough rest your body will produce larger amounts of the hunger hormone ghrelin.
This may be the reason why you are craving sweets and simple carbohydrates. Squeeze in all the rest and naps, however short, that you can.

Clean eating and weight loss

Most people will find that they lose weight quite easily when they embark on a new lifestyle of clean eating. That's generally because their bodies become more efficient – like a well-oiled Ferrari! They feel lighter, faster and stronger, because they are running on optimum fuel.

It's important to remember when you want to hit fat-loss mode, however, that even though a glorious piece of raw almond slice is nutrient dense and completely clean, you wouldn't sit down and eat five slices in one day. Raw, or clean, treats generally only contain the good fats and natural sugars, but they are a treat nevertheless. We might love a little cacao chocolate bliss ball, but if you down five in a day, you might be left not feeling so great.

Good food, but in sensible portions

You should always try to be mindful of how much you eat, especially when your goal is to lose stubborn fat. Making sure you are eating a good balance of protein, fats and carbohydrates with each meal and snack is essential, not only for weight loss but also for general good health. No matter how busy you are, eating a substantial breakfast, snack and lunch in the first half of the day will set you up for the second part of the

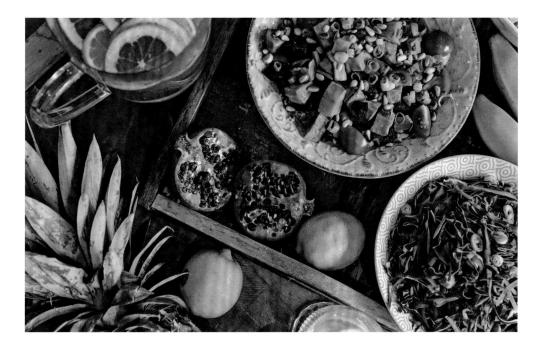

day and deter overeating in the late afternoon and night time when your activity slows down. With this in mind, try not to leave the bulk of your eating to later in the day when you are tired and less active. If you want to lose weight, clean eating doesn't mean that you eat endless amounts of food (however good it might be). You'll still need to ensure your portions are suitable and that you're including lean proteins, quality fats and carbohydrates in your diet.

Why lean proteins, quality fats and carbohydrates?

Our body needs three main nutrients in order to thrive. These nutrients are:

- Lean proteins
- Carbohydrates
- Fats

What happens when we deprive our bodies of one or more of these all-important nutrients? Well, in terms of dieting and what we put into our bodies, one of the reasons people commonly fail to succeed in maintaining a healthy diet is the tendency to restrict a major nutrient from their diet (protein, carbohydrates or fat), be it low-calorie, high protein, no carbs, shakes or an excessive amount of expensive supplements.

The problem with cutting out or severely restricting one nutrient source is that while it might work for a short period of time, it's difficult to maintain. You're more likely to experience cravings and most people end up putting the weight back on quickly – plus some more.

Starving yourself of certain nutrients can wreak havoc with your body and your mind, and this is especially so for women. Depriving yourself of wholesome proteins, carbohydrates and good fats on a daily basis can cause hormonal issues, skin problems, a lower libido, a lack of motivation and energy, anxiety and other emotional issues. All of this makes it extremely difficult to maintain any kind of diet or lifestyle change – and even more difficult to lose weight. It's also really important to be aware that going on low-calorie restrictive diets can actually increase your chances of feeling sad, anxious, worried or cranky.

On the other hand, by incorporating all three major nutrients (known as macronutrients) into your diet, you make sure that you're ticking all the boxes when it comes to what your body needs to thrive. We all need a balance of lean proteins, carbohydrates and fats in order to be healthy and happy, but which foods are rich in these essential components? Here's a quick view of the best ways to ensure you're getting enough of each in your diet.

Good sources of macronutrients

Macronutrients are the nutrients our bodies need in the largest of quantities (macro meaning large). They provide vital energy for our bodies to function efficiently in everyday life.

Protein

Animal protein*:

- Beef
- Chicken
- Eggs
- Fish and other seafood
- Lamb
- Pork
- Turkey
- Veal
- Dairy

Vegetarian protein alternatives:

- Beans and pulses/legumes that have been soaked in water before cooking
- Buckwheat
- Chia seeds
- Hemp seeds
- Quinoa
- Sunflower seeds

Carbohydrates

- Beans and legumes that have been soaked in water before cooking
- Fruit
- Vegetables
- Salad
- Whole grains (see box overleaf)

Quality fats

- Avocado
- Coconut oil
- Free-range animal products: butter, yogurt, goat's cheese
- Nuts and seeds (and relevant butters such as natural peanut butter and tahini)
- Olive oil
- Ghee

* Try to source free-range pasture-fed meats (see page 68) and dairy (see pages 51–2) . Not only do they taste better, but they also contain more antioxidants, vitamins, minerals and fatty acids and, of course, it also means that the animals involved were happier before they (or their dairy product) landed on your plate.

Which whole grains?

We have included a small amount of whole grains in our programme in the form of oats and quinoa (although strictly speaking quinoa isn't a grain, most people think of it as one). These are the two top whole grains of choice for us because they are mainly gluten-free. (See page 69 for why we aim for a mostly gluten-free lifestyle.) While oats are considered inherently gluten-free, they are frequently contaminated with wheat during their processing. So while there may be traces of gluten, they are in fact a gluten-free grain, which is why a lot of people can still tolerate them. We have limited whole grains (and most gluten) in this programme because it's important to 'clean' out your body over these four weeks and uncover which whole grains do and don't work for you. The best way to find that out is by cutting back (or if you suspect an intolerance already, eliminate them altogether) and then try re-introducing them. The majority of people find that when they cut back on these foods they experience increased energy levels, weight loss, less bloating and fewer skin problems. It's similar to the dairy scenario (see page 62).

After the four-week programme, we do recommend trialling a variety of whole grains to see how you feel on each of them. Some people may completely steer away from these foods for good, while others may find their body digests them okay.

When you wish to experiment, refer to the whole grain list below. You'll know within 30 minutes after eating the whole grains/gluten whether they sit well with you or not. If you experience instant gas, bloating, a feeling of heaviness, or find that you are holding on to excess fat on your body, it's a strong sign that your body has to work too hard to break them down.

Following the four-week programme, the best whole grains to experiment with are as follows:

- Gluten-free grains: brown rice, millet, corn, buckwheat, amaranth etc.
- If you don't suspect any intolerance at all to gluten, the best whole grains containing gluten are: wheat (remember that means the brown stuff!), rye, barley, spelt, kamut, semolina etc.

Portion sizes

Calorie counting is never fun, and with our programme it's not necessary either. When you start fuelling your body with each of these nutrients in your meals and snacks throughout the day, you'll start to notice a lot of positive changes in your energy levels, skin, fitness, waistline, patience, clarity of mind and motivation. We really aren't into calorie counting or weighing food, and our programme is jam-packed with nutrient-dense foods. All you need to do is have an idea of the way your plate should be divided up. Just visualise the picture below when preparing your meals and base your plate on these proportions. Once you begin to experience and enjoy the Stay Strong Mummy Plan for yourself, you'll be amazed at the results you get and how easy it really is.

Here's an idea of what proportions of main nutrients should make up your main meal each day. Do bear in mind that some of your fat will be contained within dressings etc.

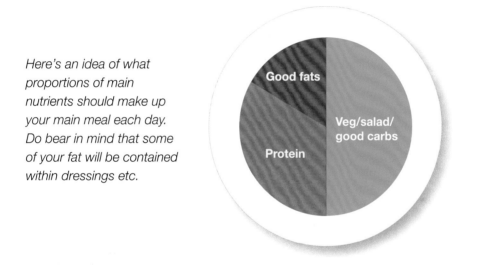

Veg/salad/good carbs Green vegetables or salad should take up half your plate, then top with colour, such as capsicum/pepper, tomatoes or other red, orange or purple vegetables and add a little starchy veg such as sweet potato, potato, celeriac, pumpkin, or squash. The starchy veg should be no bigger than the size of the palm of your hand. When using good grains, stick to the portion sizes that we have listed in each recipe.

Good fats These are quality oils such as coconut, olive, avocado, nuts, nut butter, seeds and organic butter. The *total* fats should be about half the size of your palm.

Protein Lean protein such as beef, chicken, lamb, seafood and eggs. Your protein should be about the size of the palm of your hand.

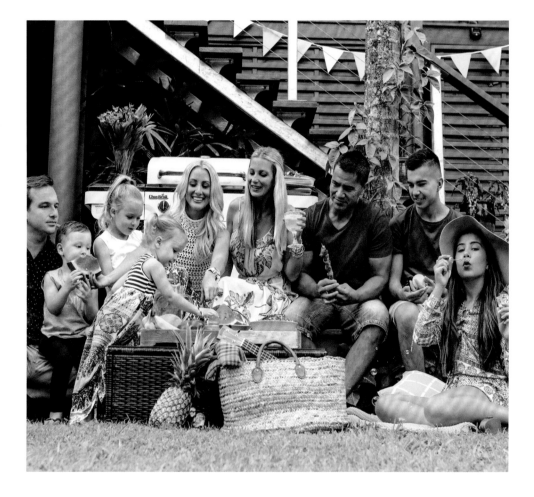

Portion sizes for the whole family

We know what you're thinking…. Do I have to cook separate meals for my husband and kids in an effort to 'lean up'? The answer is, no. However, if your hubby isn't looking to lose weight, we simply recommend serving him a bigger portion size of the same thing you are eating. For your kids' meals, increase the amount of carbohydrates to keep up with their energy levels. We also recommend adding some extra gluten-free whole grains to their meals (i.e. brown rice, gluten-free pasta). Just remember, once you get the hang of fuelling yourself and your family with clean foods, you will find your flow as the 'cook' of the family and will learn what works for all of you.

If you sense some resistance to the new foods from hubby or the kids, don't get disheartened and give up after one attempt. It can take time for their taste buds to adjust to the new flavours of real food. Let them try bits and pieces, add something new every few days and just remember, if they are super-fussy, take baby steps. Your persistence will pay off.

Healthy food comes first

Many people think that exercise is the Holy Grail for weight loss and a healthy lifestyle, but this is simply not the case. Food is your fuel, and food is your key to success. If you have had a bad night with the kids or they are unwell for a few days, you should forget the exercise altogether and just focus on your diet. Yup – you heard us right! If you've had little sleep, rather than working out, your response should be to get in the kitchen and prepare some quick but healthy snacks and meals to nourish yourself that little bit more. Putting the right food into your body will give you the boost you need to get through the day and night and to be the best mum you can be. Remember: Exercise is not the be all and end all. Healthy food is vital for success.

Stressful times are not an indication that you should throw in the towel either. When you are under stress, nourishing your body with healthy food will give you the strength to cope with what life throws at you. A bad day, bad week, or stressful situations should not be a reason for you to feel guilty because you've missed a workout or indulged in an unhealthy meal. If times do get tough, just hold your head up and remind yourself of your goals, routines and the direction you want to be heading in.

Forbidden foods

The following are the foods you should try to avoid while sticking to the plan:

- Processed and packaged foods, chips (crisps), pre-made salad dressings, frozen meals, white flours, flavoured yogurts, muesli bars, breakfast cereals, sandwich meats and condiments that contain added sweeteners, fillers and chemicals.

- Refined sugar, ice cream, lollipops, cookies, frozen drinks, chocolate bars, cakes and biscuits.

- Refined-grain white breads, pastas and white rice.

- Dairy (optional). A large number of people are intolerant to dairy. It's due to the fact that most dairy products cause inflammation in the body, insulin spikes and increased levels of mucus. Some of the most common signs of intolerance are often acne, being unable to shift excess weight, recurring sinus infections, digestive problems and bloating. However, the key is working out which type of dairy works for you and which doesn't. We have included some dairy in our guide and we recommend you opt for full-cream dairy, in the form of yogurt, goat's cheese, butter (from grass-fed cows). We don't recommend low-fat or fat-free dairy as these products have been overly processed, are often loaded with refined sugars and are devoid of all of the healthy fats. If you suspect you have an intolerance, we recommend cutting out all dairy for the four weeks and then introducing a small amount (½ cup at a time) and notice how your body reacts within 30 minutes or so of consuming it.

Tips for conscious eating

We all need reminding of the following from time to time:

- When possible, sit down to eat and be present to the moment, rather than eating to fill time.

- Minimise distractions – turn the phone, internet and TV off.

- Slow down and chew your food carefully – it's better for your digestion and you'll absorb more nutrients from your food.

- Eat until you are satisfied, not over-full.

- Always be grateful for what's on your plate, and enjoy the experience of eating.

- Use dinnertime as quality family time. Sit and talk about your day together with your family rather than eating alone and rushing through meals.

Eliminating processed foods

When you make the decision to eliminate processed foods from your diet, know that you'll need to stay emotionally strong for the first few weeks. These first few clean-eating weeks are more difficult if you've been eating sugar, wheat, dairy and commercial foods. Your body will go into detox mode and you'll be cursing our names and probably throwing this book around the room. When you do curse us, just remember that what you're going through is completely normal and, in the end, you'll feel and look awesome if you just stick with it.

'Getting through that third week of detox really is the game-changer, and if you can get through it, you've already won!'

In order to succeed, and to increase your chances of success when you're going through a detox, it will help if you put a plan in place to deal with the feelings and frustrations as they arise. Because your body has been addicted to processed foods and additives, you are likely to experience headaches, mood swings, a bad temper and feelings of overtiredness, and you are likely to give up sooner than you thought. Too much reality? Well, we're health advocates and motivators, not sales people, so we just tell it like it is so that you will know what you're in for. Trust us, it *is* worth it. Put it this way: you're better armed with reality and truth than to think that it's all too hard when you get going. You *can* do this!

How long will the frustration last once you begin your four-week Stay Strong Mummy Plan? It's likely you'll experience side effects (as above) for anything from a few days to the first two weeks, depending on the level of toxins in your body. On a brighter note though, once your detox symptoms subside, you'll notice your skin and eyes are clearer, the sugar cravings have disappeared, your body is starting to change and your energy levels are increasing. At this point you won't be cursing us anymore. Getting through that third week of detox really is the game-changer, and if you can get through it, you've already won!

Mummy Mantra

I trust my instincts

Get organised for healthy eating

Here are some top tips for detoxing your kitchen cupboards, buying wisely and saving time when prepping food:

- Detox your pantry. Throw away out-of-date and processed foods that have been bought for convenience. They don't do your body any justice.

- Make sure you have all the essential staple whole-food pantry items such as coconut oil, olive oil, almond meal (ground almonds) and coconut flour (the latter two being great gluten-free substitutes for baking or when making raw treats), raw nuts and seeds, sea salt, coconut cream and cacao powder (a healthier alternative to cocoa as it is less processed, contains no sugar and is high in antioxidants).

- Avoid packaged foods when possible.

- Shop around the outside aisles in your supermarket. Avoid the middle aisles, as these ones contain the majority of packaged processed foods. The outer aisles generally have fresh fruit, vegetables and meat products.

- Check food labels for listed ingredients. The general rule for whole-food buying is: if you can't pronounce it, don't buy it!

- Look for minimal lists of ingredients on labels: the fewer additives the better.

- Steer clear of low-fat foods. Most have added sugar, artificial sweeteners and salt to make them taste better, leaving you feeling hungrier than ever.

- When a label says 'healthy', it doesn't necessarily mean that it is. Do your own research on each food type or product, and look to find what the listed ingredients are.

- Aim for fresh produce that's in season; you'll get a good idea from visiting your local farmers' market, market or greengrocer. The bonus there is that it will be fresher and cheaper and will provide variety and inspiration at meal times. Meals are always enjoyed more when they are less repetitive.

- As soon as you buy your fruit and veg, wash, chop and put it into airtight containers in the fridge. It's then ready to go for salads, smoothies and snacks. Nothing gets wasted this way and you'll find it easier to prepare your meals.

- Make breakfast and snacks the night before. Some of the dishes that you can make the night before without compromising on taste could include a chia pudding (page 140), Overnight Oats (page 93), or a green smoothie (page 89). (Obviously a smoothie is at its nutrient-rich best if you can make it immediately before you drink it but, hey, we're realists and one that's been made the night before is still a better option than no breakfast or a less healthy alternative.)

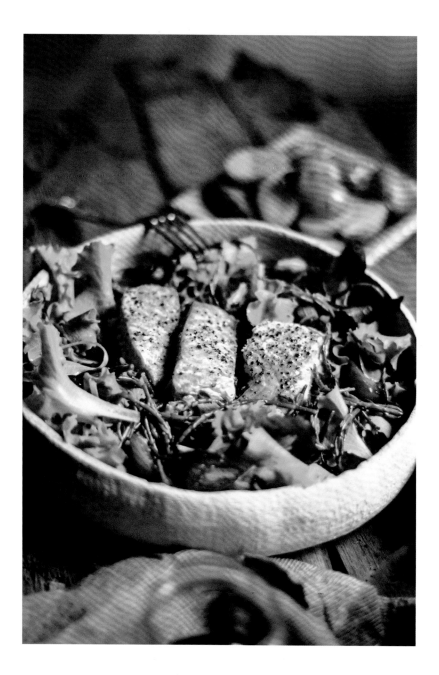

Online grocery shopping is a great alternative to shopping at your local supplier. Although we love getting to the farmers' markets now and again, the reality is that some of us can't make it there every week with the kids. Try a grocery shop online – not only will you probably find the quality, service and reliability great, but it's also proven to be very affordable. When you shop online, you know what is on your grocery list each week and can quickly search through the specials and deals. Online groceries are usually delivered within 24 hours and are fresh and on time. It's also great for mums with young babies still in nappies. You can get everything in one shop and with no hassle. Organisation is key to the Stay Strong Mummy Plan, so scheduling in your grocery shopping each week is paramount.

Protein – you need it!

You've probably heard about some of the more common diets and fads out there, but there seems to be one familiar food source that is always seen as a must have. That's protein. So what exactly is protein, and why the heck do we humans need it? We thought it would be a good idea to give you a basic rundown on what protein does for people and why it's super-important for busy mums like us.

Protein – the get up and go for humans

If we were scientists or doctors, we'd give you the following spiel: Protein is made of '... organic compounds, which have large molecules composed of ... amino acids and are an essential part of all living organisms, especially as structural components of body tissues such as muscle, hair, etc., and as enzymes and antibodies.' (From the ever-reliable Wikipedia.)

But without trying to freak you out completely by inserting too much technical stuff, here's what's so important about protein and why humans need it so much. Protein is essential for making and strengthening muscles, tendons and all organs, including your skin. Protein is crucial for normal body functions, and humans really couldn't survive without it. Often referred to as the building blocks of the human body, proteins foster human life. That is why you will note that every diet that people have ever come up with puts an emphasis on the importance of protein. And the Stay Strong Mummy Plan is no different. We want you to be strong, healthy and feelin' fine – and protein really should be one of your best friends.

Protein isn't all meat and eggs

There are many ways to get your daily requirements of protein and, of course, we'd love you to source it from whole foods, but we know that sometimes you'll need a quick protein hit, so this next section will help you decide which direction you should look to source your next protein hit. Getting all our protein from quality wholefoods is not always possible or convenient, especially when we are constantly on the go. We recommend you try to eat five servings of protein a day, and using some protein powder can be a great way to pack the protein into your daily diet.

As super-busy mums, we have at least one protein-packed green or berry smoothie every day – either as a quick and nutritious snack after a workout or for breakfast.

Please note, however, that not all protein powders are created equal. It's important to do your research and find one that is as close to nature as possible. It's great to find a good-quality whey protein isolate (from grass-fed animals – see page overleaf about quality animal produce) that is free from chemicals, fillers and artificial sweeteners. Quality protein powder plays a big part in our daily routine. It's quick and easy to incorporate into your daily meals and it's an affordable way to make sure you're getting some of what your body needs.

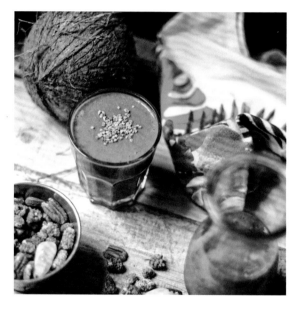

Whey protein is a dairy by-product and is a complete protein. Because whey is quickly absorbed by the body, it replenishes muscle stores depleted by workouts and everyday activity, and assists in fat loss by reducing the stress hormone cortisol while raising the feel-good hormones such as dopamine and serotonin. The added bonus is that whey helps us to feel fuller for longer by keeping our blood sugar levels stable, while helping us maintain a healthy immune system. (You'll find more about the importance of stable blood sugar on the following page.)

If you are sensitive to dairy, we recommend finding a good-quality plant-based pea protein isolate, as it has very similar qualities to whey protein isolate.

Why is stable blood sugar important for weight loss?

When you consume highly refined simple carbohydrate foods your body experiences a spike in blood sugar levels due to a rise in glucose in your bloodstream. In response to this rise in glucose levels, the pancreas releases the hormone insulin. Insulin is an anabolic hormone that's essential for getting amino acids and carbohydrates into the muscles (the amino acids promote growth and the carbohydrates provide energy).

However, when there is a pronounced blood sugar spike, your body overreacts and produces too much insulin. The insulin quickly clears the glucose from the bloodstream, leading to a sharp drop in blood sugar known as hypoglycemia.

When our blood sugar drops like this we are susceptible to sugar cravings, feelings of hunger, mood swings and lack of energy. It is a vicious cycle that can lead to more consumption of these types of foods, which will then lead to weight gain. Choosing complex carbohydrates (which release their energy more slowly) and combining them with protein and good fats, eaten every 3 hours, will ensure stable blood sugar levels and help promote weight loss.

Grass-fed, free-range and gluten-free

We mentioned earlier that it's important to make certain food choices to improve the quality of the food you eat. Here we give the reasons why animals fed naturally are beneficial to our health and why we might want to steer clear of gluten most of the time.

Grass-fed and free-range

We are both animal lovers, but other than making sure animals have a happy life before they end up on our plate, what reasons are there to select grass-fed or free-range meat for your meals?

We prefer to choose produce from these naturally reared animals firstly so that we know where our meat, eggs and dairy come from, what that animal has eaten, what kind of life it has lived (was it stressed?) and because it is always better for the animal to graze off the land rather than be restrained. But, equally importantly, we know that grass-fed and free-range animal meat is better for our bodies. This is because every cell in the human body will function better when the animal produce we eat is from naturally reared animals that have been grazing on grass or eating other natural foods. The total nutritional value of meat produced this way is increased, and these meats are also loaded with natural minerals and vitamins, which caged and grain-fed animals lack. Free-range and grass-fed animals contain five times as much CLA (conjugated linoleic acid), which has been shown to protect the heart and aid weight loss, and it is also higher in anti-inflammatory omega-3 fatty acids and vitamin D_3.

Gluten-free

It is common to find people with intolerances to food that contains gluten. But if we aren't aware of any intolerances to gluten that our body might have, why should we choose to eat gluten-free foods?

Gluten is a protein found in certain grains, such as wheat, barley, rye, spelt and semolina. Gluten not only gives baked goods their characteristic texture and chewiness, but it is also used in the processing of many other foods to add thickness, flavour and protein.

Most of us have experienced the effects of gluten, but we might not be aware that gluten was the culprit. If you eat too much gluten, it can make you feel tired and sluggish. It can also make you feel and look as if you've instantly gained weight after eating it: hello bloated tummy – where did you come from?

Gluten is extremely challenging for the body to break down, and it requires a lot of energy and a strong digestive system in order to do so. Most of us ingest far too much gluten, and so our bodies rebel, which messes with our metabolism and slows down our weight-loss progress. This is not to say that you must have a totally gluten-free diet; occasionally it feels wonderful to splurge out on a piece of freshly baked organic sourdough bread with a poached egg or a wholemeal wrap packed with a yummy salad.

If you do go gluten-free, here are some of the benefits you can expect to notice:

• Weight loss
• Reduced bloating/no bloating
• Clear skin
• Increased energy
• More positive thoughts
• Feeling lighter and more free
• Less inflammation

Now that you know our reasons for steering away from gluten and towards free-range products, what do you think about trying them yourself? It's gotta be worth a try.

Hydration – the key to losing fat

Don't underestimate the power of water. Your body is made up of approximately 70 per cent water, your brain is about 85 per cent water and your liver is 95 per cent water. Water not only carries toxins from the body, but it also transports very important water-soluble nutrients to our cells. If we could give you only one tip for your health and for fat loss, hydration would be it. Water is the first thing you should consume when you wake up in the morning – *not* tea or coffee. We know that dropping the wake-up caffeine hit is not the news you were after, but first thing in the morning is one of the most important opportunities you're presented with to flush out toxins efficiently and to get your bowels moving.

'Staying hydrated will increase your weight loss and improve your energy levels and your workouts'

We know: you've just had either an aha! moment or a pang of guilt. Right? Well, you're not alone. In fact, most of us don't drink enough water on a daily basis. So, if your excuse is that you're just too busy, or you forget to drink, then it's probably important to know that when it comes to fostering a healthy body or losing weight, by not drinking enough H_2O you really are self-sabotaging your chances of success. So let's start now – go grab a drink of water and then come back to us.

It's time to fall in love with water. We're serious. If there's one thing you can do for your health it is to stay hydrated. If you suffer from headaches, constipation, fatigue or weight gain, we guarantee water is going to be your new best friend. Your body simply cannot metabolise fat efficiently when it is dehydrated. Your liver is the organ responsible for this process. Its job is to break down the fatty acids that are metabolised into the blood stream – and it needs water to do its job properly.

How much water do we really need to drink each day? For adults, we should be aiming to drink up to 8 cups (2 litres) every day. For kids, the correct water intake depends on age and size. A rough indication would have us aim for around 3 cups (750ml) for children of 7–12 months, and for older kids up to 7 cups (1.75 litres) for 9–13-year-olds. If you live in a warmer climate or have very active kids, you might need to up your children's water intake.

As drinking ample water is a necessity in your routine – for you and your whole family – here are some things you can do to remind yourself to up the water intake. Try keeping a water bottle on your kitchen worktop or next to your desk. Set reminders on your phone to take frequent sips throughout the day and don't leave home without your water bottle.

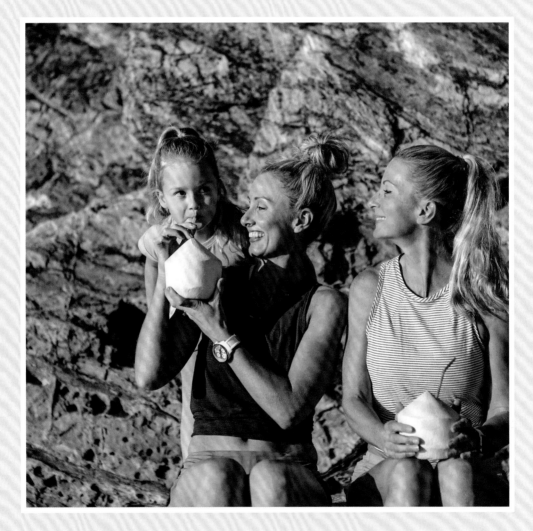

The signs of a lack of water

When we meet a client for the first time, the very first thing we will look for is the signs of fluid retention. Fluid retention shows up as a swollen face, hands, knees and feet. It's a good sign that a person is holding water, and it's usually due to dehydration. When you increase your water intake, the puffy side effects of water retention will start to disappear and you'll notice an increase in fat loss too. Although it might be inconvenient, frequent trips to the toilet are actually a good indication that you are on track to getting enough water each day.

We're not saying increasing water alone is going to help you shed kilos, but it certainly does help. And the results are maximised when combined with nutrition and exercise. Staying hydrated will increase your weight loss and improve your energy levels and your workouts.

Hydration throughout the day

The water intake our bodies need differs for each individual, due to body size and level of activity. During the Stay Strong Mummy Plan we recommend the following:

- 1–2 glasses of warm water with a slice of lemon first thing in the morning (with a dash of apple cider vinegar if you like*)
- 1 glass of water before each meal
- Build up to 8 cups a day, which equals approximately 2 litres of water (more when exercising)
- Preferably drink filtered water
- Add lemon, lime, orange, mint or strawberries to water to add flavour
- Green and herbal teas can be part of your daily quota

* A dash of apple cider vinegar in your warm lemon water every morning will assist in detoxification, digestion, alkalinity pH levels and fat loss.

Conscious coffee drinking

Coffee lovers – you're about to love us! If anyone tells you to eliminate coffee altogether, we're asking you to consider setting that advice aside. Although it's not beneficial to overdose on caffeine of any kind, coffee does have its benefits and perks. Check out our top reasons why we think coffee is more than okay in moderation.

- Coffee is high in antioxidants that can help fight free radicals in the body. Free radicals can cause Alzheimer's disease and heart disease, so a little coffee might just go a long way to keeping you healthy and helping you to keep all your marbles.

- Coffee improves mood and a sense of well-being, so a coffee a day might help you to remain calm and happy.

- Coffee improves energy and alertness, so it really can be the pick-me-up you need when concentration is necessary.

Everything in moderation

Although we might love coffee, it's important to remember that some things are best taken in moderation:

- It's important to know your limits. Tune into your body and understanding of how coffee affects you and when you've had too much.
- If you're trying to drop the pounds, avoid sugar and dairy with your coffee and opt for a black or almond milk latte instead.
- When you're feeling anxious or stressed out, try a delicious cinnamon or liquorice non-caffeinated tea instead of coffee.
- Are you using coffee to wake yourself up in the morning? It's far better to let wholesome foods do the waking and then enjoy your coffee.
- Coffee should never be used as a replacement for sleep. We need sleep to function.

Is alcohol okay?

Many of us love nothing more than to enjoy a nice glass of wine at the end of the day. Whether it's a drink with the girls or with our husbands, having a glass of wine is a wonderful ritual, and it's one that allows us to feel present with those around us and can help us to relax and unwind. We know just how good it can feel when things get crazy at home and it is finally bedtime for the kids and time for you to pop open a bottle of wine and wash the stresses of the day away with a red or white. There are, however, some considerations to be made when it comes to alcohol and staying healthy.

Alcohol and the Plan

If you have set specific goals to lose weight on the Stay Strong Mummy Plan we recommend cutting out alcohol for the whole four weeks. (Yes, four weeks!) 'But *why*?'

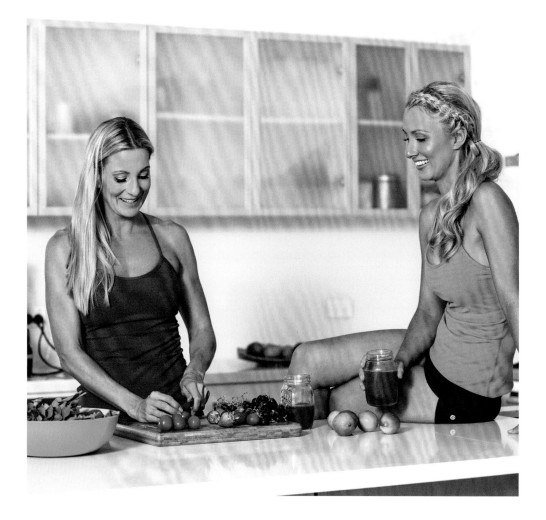

we hear you ask. If it's weight you're seeking to lose, you need to know that alcohol inhibits your body's ability to burn fat, and it can also really mess with your metabolism. Alcohol also increases your appetite and cravings for high-carbohydrate foods, which lead to weight gain.

If you're screaming under your breath while reading this, and cutting out alcohol for four weeks is not an option for you, you can always try cutting down your consumption to only one or two glasses a week. Alcohol can be part of a healthy lifestyle – both of us mummas are living proof of that! But it's always important to tune into your body and have your healthy goals in the forefront of your mind. You have to be in control here. Is the alcohol ruling you – or can you control how much alcohol you consume?

If eliminating alcohol is a big challenge for you, try replacing it with another yummy alternative. What about pouring yourself a refreshing mineral water in a wine glass with a slice of lemon? Or enjoy a glass of delicious kombucha (see page 152) while preparing the family meals?

Tips for alcohol consumption

It's easier to keep your alcohol consumption sensible if you have some strategies already in place to avoid drinking without really thinking:

- Aim to keep weekdays alcohol-free.
- Stick to one or two glasses at the weekend rather than binge drinking.
- Drink slowly and enjoy the experience.
- Avoid alcohol during periods when you're actively trying to lose body fat (and not simply maintaining a steady weight).
- Fill up on a smoothie (pages 89 and 90) before you go out to social gatherings to help avoid the desire to revert to unhealthy nibbles and alcohol.
- Find some alternative drinks that you like, or drink water instead of alcohol.
- Try wine and soda water or carbonated water as a spritzer.

Your healthy-option meal plan

To make your transition into clean eating easier, and to ensure you stay on track, we've taken the hard work out of it for you and created a meal plan based on what we both eat ourselves. It is a two-week plan and includes some of our favourite meals to give you a realistic, delicious menu so that you can focus on eating well and feeling great. All the meals can be found in our recipe section in Chapter 5.

The protein component for each recipe can be swapped around to suit your preference; for example, red meat can be substituted with chicken or fish. Take a look at our carefully crafted meal plan and see what tickles your taste buds.

Eating from the Stay Strong Mummy meal plan will ensure that you feel satisfied, healthy and vitalised. And while you're at it, you'll notice your waistline and your grocery-shopping bill shrinking too.

We have carefully crafted every meal you'll need in our four-week programme. Breakfast, lunch, dinner, snacks and optional sweet treats are all listed, so you don't have to worry about what to eat or when. As this is a two-week plan, you simply repeat it to cover the four weeks.

Alternatively, you may wish to put together your own meal plans, in which case use the menu choices given on pages 79–82. You create your own menu by selecting three meals and two snacks from the options to make up your own daily menu. You can choose to vary each day or eat the bulk of the same foods for one week and mix it up the next. It's up to you.

Stick to the principles

Eating regularly is important for health and vitality. Skipping meals, on the other hand, is detrimental to your health. If you can get your diet right by eating clean, whole foods every three hours and making sure you include the three macronutrients (lean proteins, quality fats and carbohydrates) *and* if you genuinely commit to following this programme for four weeks, we know that you will see awesome results and feel amazing – just like we did.

With the Stay Strong Mummy Plan, there's no need to be scared of exercise or food preparation, and there is no need to wonder anymore if you can succeed with your weight loss and health-and-fitness goals. If you follow our guidelines, implement the meal plans that we've created for you and commit to this programme, you *will* be successful, because the recipe for success is 80 per cent diet and only 20 per cent exercise.

Gone are the days when you spend your money on expensive pre-packaged foods that leave you feeling empty or when you throw away food that nobody bothered to eat. It's time for a fresh start, and we're here to help you get it right.

Tip: When to eat

Schedule your HIIT/exercise (see Chapter 6) before a high-protein smoothie snack or meal for optimal muscle recovery and repair.

Our sample menu plan – week 1

	Monday	Tuesday	Wednesday	Thursday	Friday	Saturday	Sunday
Upon waking	Warm water with lemon and apple cider vinegar	Warm water with lemon and apple cider vinegar	Warm water with lemon and apple cider vinegar	Warm water with lemon and apple cider vinegar	Warm water with lemon and apple cider vinegar	Warm water with lemon and apple cider vinegar	Warm water with lemon and apple cider vinegar
Breakfast	Perfect Green Smoothie Black coffee or tea	Easy-As Vegetable Omelette Black coffee or tea	Overnight Oats topped with ¼ cup fruit Black coffee or tea	Perfect Green Smoothie Black coffee or tea	Classy Apple Cinnamon Bircher Black coffee or tea	Scrambled Eggs, Bacon and Avocado Treat Black coffee or tea	Pancakes with Punch Black coffee or tea
Snack	2 boiled eggs and 1 cup raw vegetables e.g. carrot, celery, cucumber	Perfect Green Smoothie	1 apple with 1 tbsp natural nut butter	1 boiled egg and ½ cup cashews	2 stalks celery with 2 tbsp natural nut butter	Berry Protein Smoothie	Perfect Green Smoothie
Lunch	Crunchy Kale and Chickpea Salad served with chicken or tuna for extra protein	Baked Salmon and Green Salad	Rainbow Rice Paper Rolls served with chicken for added protein, and green salad	Bacon and Cauliflower Rice Bowl	Egg, Pear and Walnut Salad	Rainbow Tuna Salad	Leftover Warm Quinoa and Halloumi Salad
Snack	Small handful of almonds, ½ cup strawberries, 1 tbsp of full-fat Greek yogurt	1 cup berries, 1–2 tbsp coconut cream sprinkled with cinnamon*	Perfect Green Smoothie	Strawberry Chia Pudding	Berry Protein Smoothie	1 apple with 1 tbsp natural nut butter	Small handful of almonds, ½ cup strawberries, 1 tbsp full-fat Greek yogurt
Dinner	Gourmet Meat Patties	Chicken and Tumeric Casserole	Beef Stir-Fry	Mexican Mince Lettuce Cups	Stuffed Sweet Potato with Creamy Avocado Dressing	Warm Quinoa and Halloumi Salad served with beef or chicken kebabs for added protein	Caramelised Onion Pizza

*Optional – protein powder mixed in

Our sample menu plan – week 2

	Monday	Tuesday	Wednesday	Thursday	Friday	Saturday	Sunday
Upon waking	Warm water with lemon and apple cider vinegar	Warm water with lemon and apple cider vinegar	Warm water with lemon and apple cider vinegar	Warm water with lemon and apple cider vinegar	Warm water with lemon and apple cider vinegar	Warm water with lemon and apple cider vinegar	Warm water with lemon and apple cider vinegar
Breakfast	Perfect Green Smoothie Black coffee or tea	Overnight Oats topped with ¼ cup fruit Black coffee or tea	Scrambled Eggs, Bacon and Avocado Treat Black coffee or tea	Berry Protein Smoothie Black coffee or tea	Easy-As Vegetable Omelette Black coffee or tea	Pancakes with Punch Black coffee or tea	Classy Cinnamon Bircher Black coffee or tea
Snack	2 boiled eggs and 1 cup raw vegetables e.g. carrot, celery, cucumber	Perfect Green Smoothie	Berry Protein Smoothie	1 boiled egg and ½ cup cashews	1 apple with 1 tbsp natural nut butter	Perfect Green Smoothie	Small handful of almonds, ½ cup strawberries and 1 tbsp full-fat Greek yogurt
Lunch	Rainbow Rolls with tuna or chicken on the side	Sweet Potato and Zucchini Frittata	Crunchy Kale and Chickpea Salad	Bacon and Cauliflower Rice Bowl	Egg, Pear and Walnut Salad	Leftover Lamb Shank Vegetable Soup	Baked Salmon and Green Salad
Snack	Small handful of almonds, ½ cup strawberries and 1 tbsp full-fat Greek yogurt	1 boiled egg and ½ cup cashews	1 apple with 1 tbsp natural nut butter	Berry Protein Smoothie	1 cup berries, 1–2 tbsp coconut cream sprinkled with cinnamon*	Strawberry Chia Pudding	Perfect Green Smoothie
Dinner	Beef Stir-Fry	Chicken and Zucchini Noodles with Creamy Basil Sauce	Spiced Barbecue Steak and Jacket Potato with green salad	Sweet Potato Curry with Prawns	Lamb Shank Vegetable Soup	Bacon and Mushroom Frittata	Almond-Coated Chicken with Red Cabbage Coleslaw

*Optional – protein powder mixed in

Choosing your own menu

On the following pages you will find a list of all our recipes to help you put together your own menu plan.

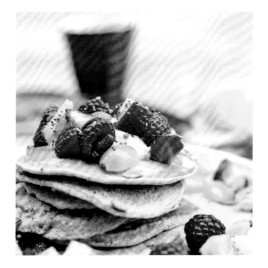

Breakfasts

Morning Glory – Perfect Green Smoothie (page 89)

Berry Protein Smoothie (page 90)

Scrambled Eggs, Bacon and Avocado Treat (page 91)

Overnight Oats (page 93)

Classy Apple Cinnamon Bircher (page 94)

Pancakes with Punch (page 96)

Easy-As Vegetable Omelette (page 99)

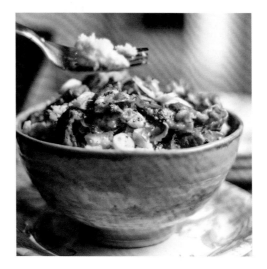

Lunches

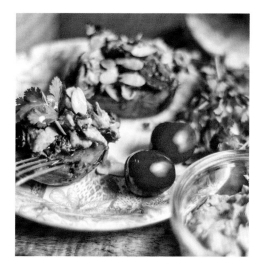

Dinners

Snacks

It is important not to get too hungry so it is fine to have two snacks a day.

2 hard-boiled eggs, plus 1 cup (1 handful) raw vegetables

1 small handful of almonds, plus ½ cup (100g) strawberries or berries and
1 tbsp full-fat Greek yogurt

1 cup (100g) berries (fresh or frozen) topped with 1–2 tbsp coconut cream and
sprinkled with cinnamon, plus 1 scoop natural protein powder (optional)

1 apple with 1 tbsp natural nut butter

Sweet treats

If you feel your resolve slipping and you're tempted to reach for the biscuit jar, then
these recipes are a great back-up. We would rather you snack on one of these
healthier treats than a refined sugar treat. If you're trying to lose weight, stick to one
to two of these treats per week.

Strawberry Chia Pudding (page 140)

Mango Maca Protein Smoothie (page 143)

Almond Mocha Smoothie (page 144)

Cashew, Coconut and Lemon Protein Balls (page 147)

Simply Raw Choc Almond Slice (page 148)

Sides for immunity and gut health

Bone Broth (made with beef or chicken) (page 151)

Kombucha (page 152)

A focus on fat loss – and what carbs have to do with it

If you are finding it difficult to drop body fat, you are not alone. Stubborn body fat is one of the most talked about subjects in the Stay Strong Mummy community. Unfortunately, for us women, our bodies don't make the process of burning fat easy. The female body prefers to burn carbohydrates as fuel – and that means fat-burning comes second.

When you remove processed carbohydrates from your diet, generally you will lose weight; however, for most people, cutting out all carbohydrates will leave you feeling flat and usually craving carbs more than ever. It is common for those who have tried a no-carb diet to quickly find out that it's not enjoyable or sustainable. After a brief period of depriving their bodies, they usually end up putting all of the weight back on, and more. The fact is this way of eating simply doesn't contribute to a well-balanced and realistic diet for you and your family.

Healthy carbs versus non-healthy carbs

It is important to understand the difference between healthy carbs (complex carbs) and non-healthy carbs (simple carbs).

Healthy carbohydrates are the foods that are still in their natural state or have gone through minimal processing. These are the carbohydrates that we list on pages 58–9. Think fruit, starchy vegetables and whole grains. They release their energy slowly into the body, which helps stabilise your blood sugar, ensuring an even, lasting energy level. When your energy levels are stable, you don't have those 10am and 3pm crash hours when you're starving and needing those biscuits just to get you through to the next meal (hence, weight gain).

Non-healthy carbohydrates are foods that have been refined. Think white rice, white bread, white pasta, packet noodles, and so on. Most of the time, these foods have been stripped of their nutrients, are sometimes bleached to radiate that white, shiny colour and all you are left with is a nutrient-sparse carb that will send your blood sugar levels crazy (see page 68 for more about blood sugar levels). Do you ever wonder why you can eat an entire bowl of pasta or a big sandwich and feel full for 30 minutes, and then you're looking at the clock wondering when the next meal is coming? This style of carbohydrates wreaks havoc with your body (and mind). When you choose the right carbs, however, you can still have them as part of a balanced diet and lose weight. The key is to ensure that they are portioned correctly and eaten with lean protein and some good fat.

Fat-loss tips

Here, in a nutshell, is what we advise in order to achieve your fat-loss goals:

- Stick to our programme.
- Nutrition needs to be your priority, eliminating processed foods and sugary drinks.
- Focus on whole foods with high-nutrient-value quality protein, carbohydrates and good fats.
- Planning and preparation are going to be your keys to success.
- Always eat at regular intervals, be aware of hunger cues, feel satisfied not full. Aim for three meals and two snacks every day.
- Never skip breakfast! You need it to kick-start your metabolism.
- Write a food diary to keep track of what's working and what's not working.
- Include a good source of protein with every meal to help you feel fuller for longer and to reduce cravings.
- Don't overeat at night. And no snacking after dinner. Break the habit by sipping green or herbal tea.
- Keep your portions in check – if you are not looking forward to each meal and snack, you may have overeaten.
- Drink at least 8 cups (2 litres) of water a day.
- Limit or cut out alcohol if you are not losing body fat.
- Incorporate at least three workouts into your week, including HIIT and strength training (see Chapter 6). Mix up your workouts, because the more efficient you become the harder it will be to drop body fat. This is why we love HIIT – short uncomfortable bursts!
- Try to get quality rest and time to de-stress: try walking, yoga, meditation.
- Ask for support and help from online groups and forums.
- Have a clear vision of what you want to achieve, visualise it, write it down and feel it.

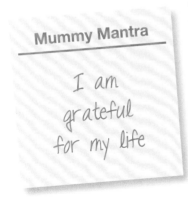

Mummy Mantra

I am grateful for my life

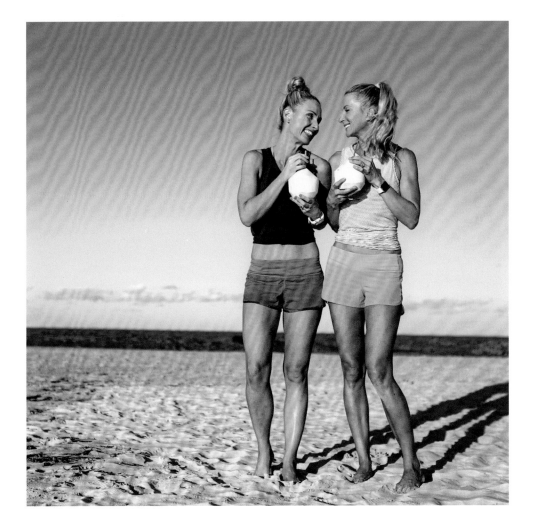

CHAPTER 5

The Recipes

When thinking about what to cook each day we like to keep it really simple by building each meal around a source of quality protein, then adding our vegetables, quality carbohydrates, and fats to the mix. Do remember that when buying meat and animal produce (eggs, dairy and meat), you should go for free-range and grass-fed wherever possible (as explained on page 68), and preferably organic.

It's important not to get overwhelmed and over-complicate the important task of nourishing yourself and your family. When you start writing out your shopping list and organising your meal plan you will notice that we use similar ingredients in many of our recipes, for example eggs, sweet potato and leafy greens. This is because:

- The whole family likes them, which means no separate meals for kids or partners.
- They have awesome nutritional and health benefits.
- They are cost-effective – a little goes a long way and there is rarely any waste.
- They are versatile.
- They can be stored in the fridge or freezer.

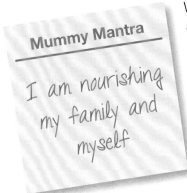

Mummy Mantra

I am nourishing my family and myself

We understand that everyone's tastes will vary from time to time, and that family members may have intolerances or allergies to certain foods. However, the fantastic thing about cooking with whole foods is that there is always an alternative. Don't be afraid to experiment with our recipes, changing things to suit your household.

Breakfasts for mums on the go

It's no secret that breakfast is the most important meal of the day, especially when we are trying to lose weight. The word 'breakfast' originally came from the term 'break fast', meaning that it's time to break the overnight fast and eat again. When our mornings are super-busy, it can be easy to forget that our last meal might have been close to 12 hours ago. By the time morning comes, your body is waiting for nourishment. If you skip breakfast, your body will go into starvation mode and start holding onto any fat stores you might have and, as a result, your metabolism will slow down, making it very difficult for your body to lose weight.

If breakfast is the most important meal of the day, shouldn't your breakfast be delicious, nourishing and enjoyable? Okay, okay, we know exactly what you're thinking: you don't have time, the house is hectic in the morning and, when you first get up and running in the morning, you're not inspired to get cracking in the kitchen. How can you possibly get inspired in the kitchen *and* make it out the door on time? We really do understand that mornings can be rushed and chaotic, especially when you're dealing with fussy eaters, a lost shoe and you're running on little sleep.

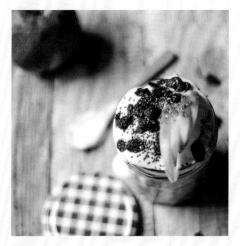

One way to ensure you get through the morning chaos and still get the nutrients you and your busy family need is to prepare your breakfast meals the night before. Our meal plan has some cook-on-the-spot meals and also some you can get ready at night to make your mornings a little less stressful. These quick-and-easy breakfast recipes present the perfect opportunity to fuel your body and begin your day on the right foot. We love these high-protein, slow-energy-release carbohydrate breakfasts, and we know they will help you to feel fuller for longer, plus they will get you through a busy morning and will replenish you after a workout.

If you like the sound of adding an extra boost to these perfectly yummy breakfast recipes, you can try adding some protein powder. (If you do add protein powder, just add a dash of water so that your meal isn't too dry.)

We've taken the stress out of helping you get breakfast just right, so that you can set the tone for an awesome day. Check out these delicious brekky-on-the-go recipes that will make sure you balance the nutrients your body needs with the yum factor we know you'll love.

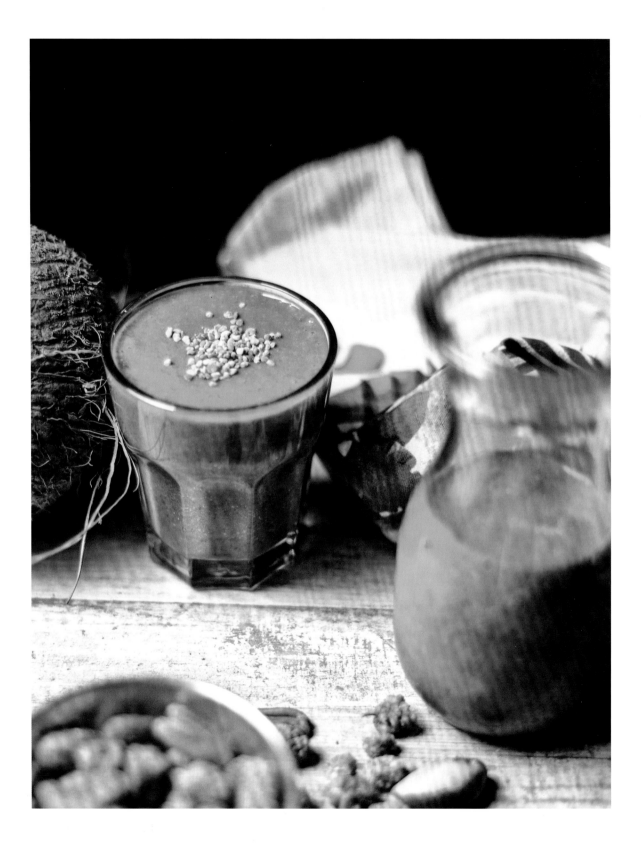

Morning Glory – Perfect Green Smoothie

We know how busy you are. But seriously, it's so essential that you nourish your body to get through this new day. Whip up this smoothie and you'll feel far more able to cope. Trust us – this one is good! Bee pollen is a subtle, sweet immune-boosting superfood and we often sprinkle it on our smoothies.

What's in it?

- 1 scoop natural protein powder
- ½ banana, sliced and frozen
- ½ cup (a small handful) dark leafy greens
- 1 thumbnail-sized piece of root ginger
- 1 tsp ground cinnamon
- 2 cups (500ml) coconut water or filtered water
- 1–2 cups (1 handful) ice, to taste
- 1 tsp raw honey (optional)

Put all the ingredients into a blender or food processor and blitz until smooth. It's really that simple. No need to worry about the order or the prep, just throw it in, blitz and enjoy!

Tips

To make life easier and to speed up your smoothie prep, bananas can be peeled, chopped and stored in the freezer until you get that smoothie craving. Using frozen banana saves time and gives your morning smoothie an ice-cold kick that you'll love to run out the door with.

If you have a hectic morning on the horizon and you just don't think you'll have time to whizz up a Morning Glory, you can always blitz it the night before and store it in the fridge for the next morning.

Berry Protein Smoothie

Most people love smoothies. We don't really have to say too much about this one, because it's just that good and a real crowd pleaser – kids love it too.

SERVES 1

What's in it?

1 cup (1 large handful) ice

1 cup (130g) frozen mixed berries

½ banana, sliced

½ cup (1 small handful) spinach

1–2 cups (250–500ml) non-sweetened almond milk, to taste

1 scoop natural protein powder

Put all the ingredients into a blender or food processor. Put the lid on and blitz until well mixed. Serve.

Tips

All of our recipes are specially designed for busy mums on the go. We make sure that these meals have just what you need to thrive and feel great. But if you have other healthy ingredients to hand and you really want to add them, go ahead. Remember: it's for you. Sometimes we also add a little more of one or other ingredient, depending on our mood. See what you think, and add more if you prefer.

If you're not a fan of almond milk, try substituting with filtered water and adding 1 tbsp full-fat Greek yogurt to give an extra hit of creaminess and protein.

Scrambled Eggs, Bacon and Avocado Treat

Who said that whole-food eating couldn't include a little bacon? For all the bacon-and-egg lovers out there, this one is for you. Enjoy! And remember that free-range and pasture-fed is best. You'll notice that eggs are a big part of our diet. Why? Because they are high in protein, vitamins and minerals, and they're inexpensive. The options are endless when whipping up a quick snack of egg-something. Adding your favourite ingredients to the mix, such as tasty bacon and avocado (which contains good fats), will leave you feeling full and satisfied.

SERVES 1

What's in it?

1 tsp coconut oil

2 bacon rashers (nitrate-free)

1 tsp butter

2 medium eggs

1 spring onion, chopped

6 cherry tomatoes, sliced

¼ avocado, chopped

Heat the coconut oil in a frying pan over a medium heat and add the bacon rashers. Cook on both sides until crispy. Remove from pan and leave on a paper towel to drain the excess oil and fat.

Heat the butter in a separate frying pan over a medium heat. Whisk the eggs and add them to the frying pan. As they start to set, stir them with a wooden spoon to scramble them.

Drain the excess fat from the frying pan used to cook the bacon, and add the spring onion and cherry tomatoes, then cook for 2 minutes or until softened. Serve the eggs with the bacon, cooked vegetables and avocado.

Tips

Piggies are important to us. When we eat bacon, we always make sure its free-range, aka: previously happy bacon. It's just another way that we can have a positive impact on our world and environment.

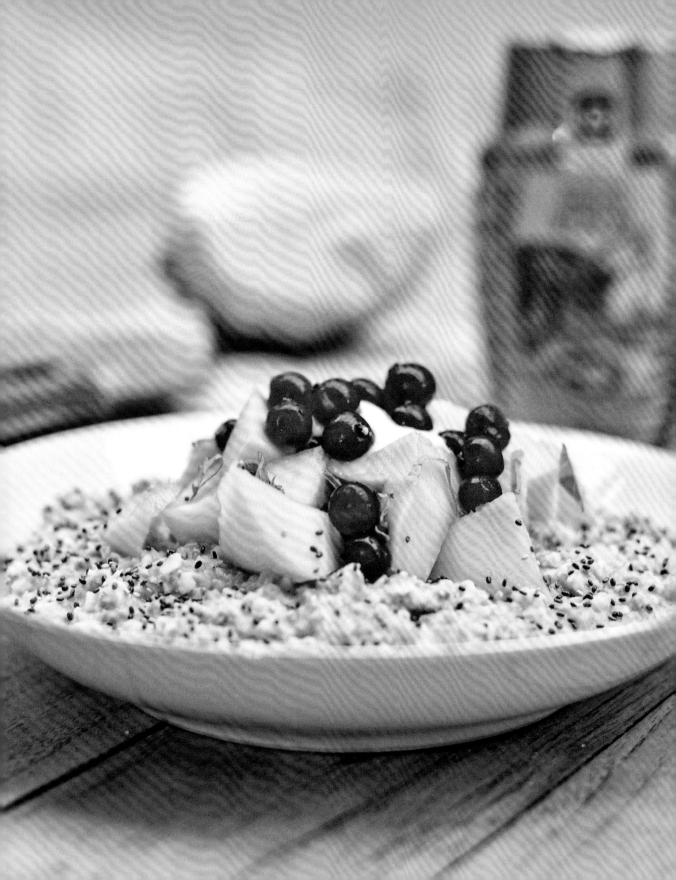

Overnight Oats

Cooking your breakfast the night before? Yes! This quick whip-up will knock the socks off instant oats any day. It's simple, nutritious, yummy and easy-peasy. Oh, and did we mention it's another great Stay Strong Mummy quickie? Beware – the kids are sure to want to eat this right off your plate. These perfect winter-warmer oats will save you time if you make a few bowls in advance and store them in the fridge for up to 3–4 days.

SERVES 1

What's in it?

¼ cup (25g) rolled oats

2 tsp chia seeds

1 cup (25ml) filtered water or nut milk of choice, plus extra if needed

Topping

½ cup (110g) sliced mango and pomegranate or other fruit in season

1 tbsp full-fat Greek or coconut yogurt

1 tsp raw honey (optional)

Put the oats in a small bowl and add the chia seeds and water. Stir well, then pop it in the fridge until you're ready to eat it the next day.

When the sun's up and you're ready to devour your Overnight Oats, all that's left to do is heat it and add the topping. For convenient and quick heating, you can microwave at Full Power for approximately 1 minute or put it in a small saucepan over a medium heat for 5 minutes or until heated through, stirring occasionally. Once warm, stir in more water or nut milk if you want to make the mixture a little runnier. Then it's time to add the toppings and enjoy.

Tips

If you're sensitive to gluten, you can use gluten-free oats or substitute quinoa flakes for the oats.

If this recipe tickles your fancy, or the kids want to eat yours, you can simply double the ingredients and make enough for a few days – or for more people.

Classy Apple Cinnamon Bircher

We love this recipe. A step up from Overnight Oats, Classy Apple Cinnamon Bircher is a regular on fancy-restaurant brekky menus and a must-add to your morning pampering. Bircher is not only great for breakfast, but it's also the perfect snack, because it's quick and very easy to make. Make it in advance, pour it into jars and store in the fridge. Top with a little cinnamon to help balance out the sugars in the fruit and to boost your metabolism.

SERVES 1

What's in it?

¼ cup (25g) rolled oats

1 apple, chopped

1 tbsp raisins (preservative-free)

2 tsp chia seeds

2 tsp ground cinnamon

1 cup (250ml) almond milk, plus extra if needed

Topping

1 tbsp full-fat Greek yogurt or coconut yogurt

1 tsp raisins

1 tsp raw honey (optional)

Put the oats, apple, raisins, chia seeds and cinnamon in a bowl or container and cover with the milk. Pop it in the fridge overnight or until you're ready to devour it.

When you're ready to gobble this awesome brekky, all that's left to do is to add your toppings and enjoy. No heating, no mixing – just yummo!

Tips

If you're sensitive to gluten, you can replace rolled oats with gluten-free oats or quinoa flakes.

This dish is just as nice served warm. Heat it up in a small saucepan over a medium heat (or in a microwave on Full Power) until warmed through, approximately 1–2 minutes.

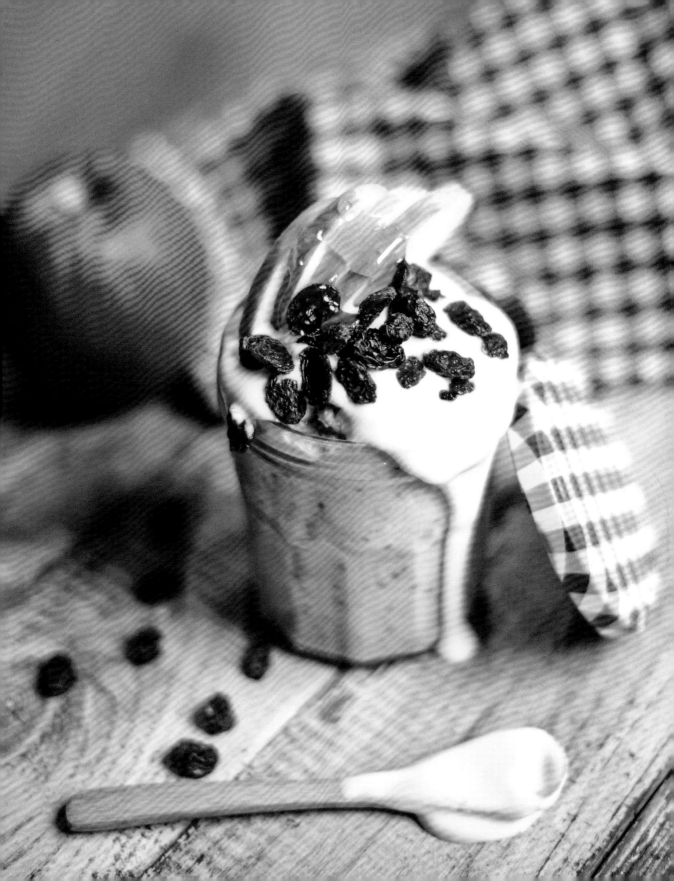

Pancakes with Punch

Who doesn't love pancakes for breakfast? We've decided that we all deserve pancakes more than just on our birthdays or Mother's Day. So we've come up with a guilt-free recipe for protein pancakes, so that you can get your protein hit as well as a touch of pampering. Pancake Sunday has long been a tradition in our households. The kids sit up at the kitchen bench (yes, even our teenagers) waiting patiently while the smell wafts through the house. Naturally sweet, gluten-free and high in protein, these healthier versions are jam-packed with goodness that the whole family can enjoy.

SERVES 1

What's in it?

1 ripe banana

2 medium eggs

¼ cup (35g) natural protein powder

1 tsp coconut oil

Topping

1 tbsp coconut cream (chilled in the fridge overnight)

½ banana or ½ cup seasonal berries or favourite fruit

2 tsp natural maple syrup

In a bowl, mash the banana with the eggs and protein powder until you get a smooth consistency. (Forget the flour – this is your new favourite pancake mix.)

Heat the oil in a non-stick frying pan over a medium-high heat. (There's nothing more frustrating than ugly pancakes that refuse to come off the pan.) Pour ¼ cup (60ml) of your pancake mixture into the hot pan.

Reduce the heat to medium and cook each pancake for 2–3 minutes or until the pancake is golden brown on the underside. Flip the pancake and cook until other side is also golden and irresistible.

When cooked, put the pancake to one side and continue with the remaining mixture until all the pancakes are cooked. And then – the best part – add the toppings and serve.

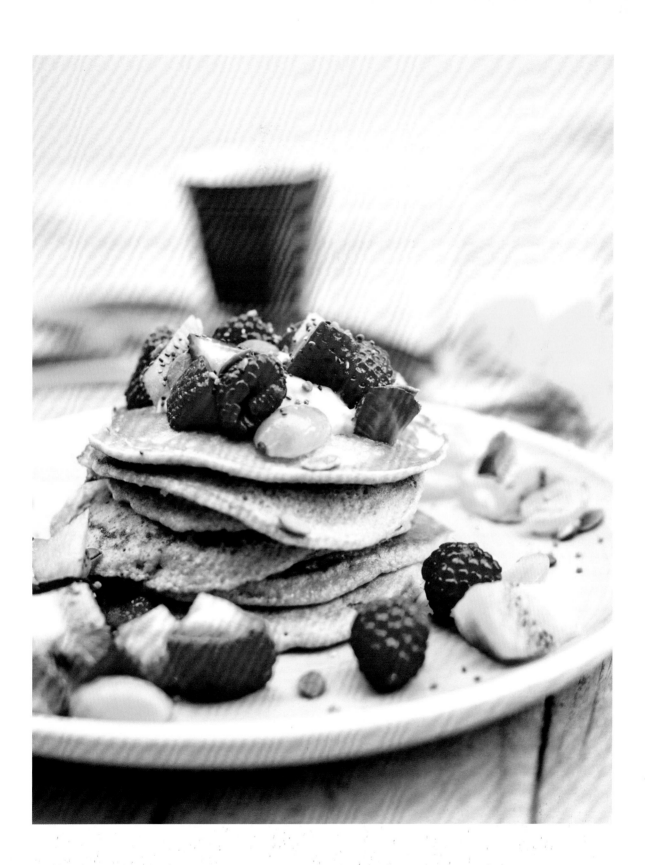

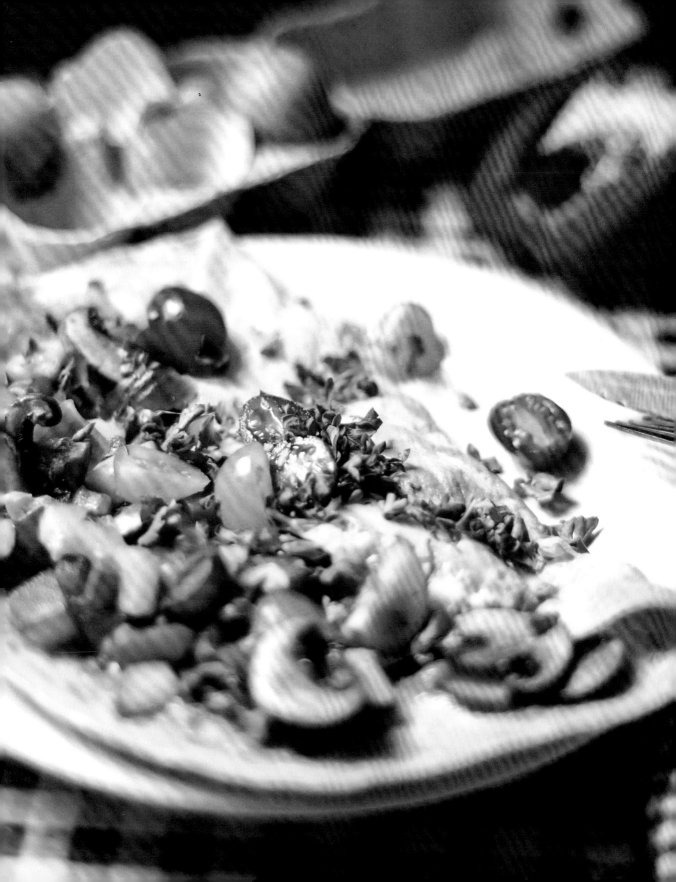

Easy-As Vegetable Omelette

If you think an omelette is too time-consuming for your morning schedule, think again. Eggs are high in protein and are the perfect way to start your day if long-lasting energy is what you need. This omlette hits the spot when it comes to a nutrient-dense meal packed with vegetables and high in protein. It's always a good idea to have your vegetables prewashed, chopped, stored in the fridge and ready to go.

SERVES 1

What's in it?

1 tbsp coconut oil, butter or ghee

½ red onion, finely chopped

3–4 mushrooms, finely chopped

1 cup (170g) cherry tomatoes, finely chopped

1 cup (1 large handful) mixed vegetables, such as spinach, zucchini (courgette), capsicum (pepper), finely chopped

2 medium eggs

sea salt and ground black pepper

chopped fresh herbs, to sprinkle

Heat half of the oil in a frying pan over a medium heat and add the vegetables. Cook for 5–10 minutes until the onion is transparent and the vegetables have softened. Set the vegetables aside.

Whisk the eggs in a bowl. Heat the remaining oil in the frying pan and add the eggs, tipping the pan to spread them evenly. Leave to cook for 5 minutes or until the eggs are partially cooked. Add the vegetables to one-half of the omelette. Leave to continue cooking. When fully cooked, gently flip the plain half of the omelette over the veggie-covered half. Slide the omelette onto a plate and season with salt and pepper, then sprinkle over some herbs.

What a great way to get in a serving of fresh veggies and protein.

Tips

We always choose free-range hens' eggs over caged or barn eggs. Why? Because it's been scientifically proven that happy chickens lay better eggs. Plus, we like to envisage our chooks running, pecking and frolicking before we take their precious eggs and eat 'em!

Lunches for ladies on a mission

Too often lunch meals are missed or replaced with snacks and nibbles throughout the day. This is especially so for those working long hours, stay-at-home parents and people under stress. Missing meals sends the body into panic and signals our internal systems to begin storing fat. Obviously, this is not a great scenario for those of us looking to lose weight or get healthy.

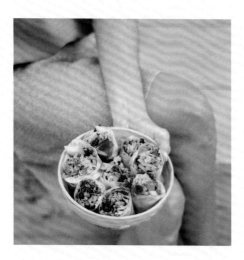

Lunch is often underrated when it comes to creating a healthy nutritional balance, and busy lifestyles can lead to a compromise on both nutrition and taste. We know that there are loads of busy mummas out there who skip lunch, but it's time to stop and think about what's best for you. After all, how can you expect to support a growing family if you don't ensure your own health and vitality first?

Eating a good-sized lunch with a quality source of protein and an abundance of salad or vegetables is crucial to staying energised and to stop you bingeing on junk foods, but, most importantly, it will reduce the urge to overeat at night time (eat well at lunchtime and say goodbye to the night-time munchies).

The sure-fire way to make sure you have a balanced lunch is to prepare your meals in advance. Carrots can be grated, lettuce leaves washed, vegetables washed and chopped, and meat for lunch the next day can be cooked the night before when you are preparing your dinner.

Leftover food from dinner is the perfect time-saver for the next day's lunch, so it's handy to keep this in mind when preparing dinner and then cooking a few extra vegetables or an extra piece of meat.

Here's a perfectly balanced lunch menu – crafted just for you!

Sweet Potato and Zucchini Frittata

Frittatas are a staple in our homes because they are a fantastic food to eat on the go, and they can be eaten for breakfast, lunch or dinner. Plus, they keep well in the fridge and can be eaten hot or cold. Any vegetable can be thrown in, which means lots of flavour combinations and less waste. This is one of our most famous Stay Strong Mummy sweet potato recipes. We use sweet potato a lot in our dishes, not only because of the sweet taste and versatility of this very cool veggie, but also because it's such a nutritionally dense superfood. It is high in protein, making it good for helping to repair cells, and it also acts as an anti-inflammatory. Sweet potato (also known as kumara) is high in fibre, helping us to feel fuller for longer. It is also jammed with vitamins A and E to protect our bodies from free radicals that damage cells.

SERVES 4

What's in it?

- 1 tbsp coconut oil, melted, plus extra for greasing
- 2 cups (230g) peeled and diced sweet potato
- 1 tsp dried basil or mixed herbs
- 8 medium eggs
- 1 large zucchini (courgette), grated
- ¼ cup (30g) diced goat's cheese
- sea salt and ground black pepper

Preheat the oven to 170°C/325°F/gas 3. Line a baking tin with baking paper and grease with a little coconut oil. Put the sweet potato in a large bowl and add the oil. Add the herbs, and stir to coat. Season with salt and pepper. Spread the sweet potato evenly over the prepared baking tin and bake for 30–40 minutes until soft in the middle and crispy on the outside. Set aside to cool.

Meanwhile, whisk the eggs in a large bowl and stir in the zucchini. Season with salt and pepper. Gently pour on top of the potatoes in the baking tray and spread out evenly, then top with the goat's cheese. Cook in the oven for 20 minutes or until cooked in the centre. Remove from the oven and serve warm or cold.

Tips

Be careful not to over-bake the frittata.

You can add bacon and extra vegetables, if you like.

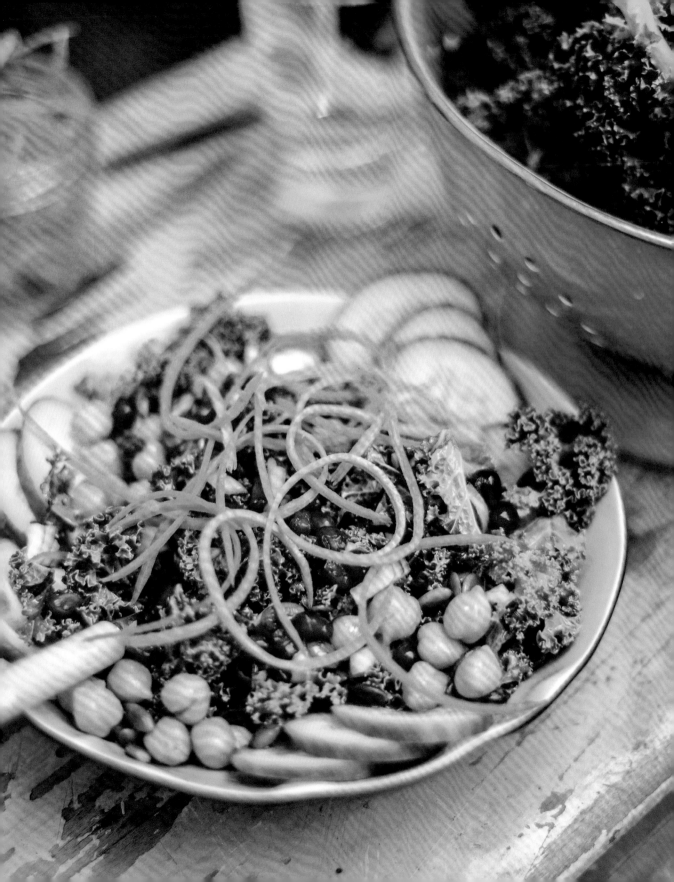

Crunchy Kale and Chickpea Salad

This salad is nourishing and has an amazing flavour burst that you just wouldn't expect. Chickpeas make for a great protein boost to any salad; they're an inexpensive meat alternative and are full of fibre and nutrients. This easy salad can be prepped in advance if you like: wash and chop the kale, then store in the fridge, grate the carrot and toast those yummy sunflower seeds (more essential fatty acids) and you'll save yourself a bundle of time. This salad complements any meat dish.

SERVES 1

What's in it?

2 cups (2 large handfuls) finely chopped kale

¼ cup (40g) drained canned chickpeas (organic), rinsed

¼ small red onion, sliced

½ small carrot, grated

½ small cucumber, chopped

¼ avocado, sliced

½ cup (60g) sunflower seeds, lightly toasted in a dry frying pan

¼ pomegranate (optional)

Dressing

1 tbsp extra virgin olive oil

1 tsp apple cider vinegar

1 tbsp tahini

sea salt and ground black pepper

Put the dressing ingredients into a screwtop jar and shake until well mixed. Place the kale in a bowl, add the dressing and, using your hands, gently massage the dressing into the leaves. Now add the chickpeas, onion, carrot, cucumber and avocado and mix everything together well. Top with toasted sunflower seeds and pomegranate, if using.

Tips

Add chicken or tuna for extra protein.

If you sprinkle some lemon juice over your pre-grated carrot, it will stop it from turning brown.

Kale is full of phytonutrients, but it can be a little tart and hard on the digestion when eaten raw. By rubbing the oily dressing into its leaves you soften the texture and the taste, and you also make the nutrients easier to absorb.

You can use pepitas (pumpkin seeds) instead of sunflower seeds.

Quick and Easy Ham and Salad Wrap

Some days, there's nothing like a ham and salad sandwich to hit the spot. For a lighter version that still does the trick, try this version, which uses lettuce leaves instead of a tortilla.

SERVES 1

What's in it?

2 large Iceberg lettuce leaves

2 slices good-quality ham

1 handful of fresh spinach leaves and alfalfa

1 small carrot, grated

1 small raw beetroot, grated

sliced tomato and cucumber

¼ avocado, mashed

1 tsp mustard

Place the lettuce leaves on a plate, and spread evenly with the avocado and mustard. Layer with the ham, spinach, alfalfa, carrot, beetroot and sliced tomato and cucumber. Gently roll into a wrap and enjoy the crunch.

Tips

Good quality free-range ham isn't always easy to find. You may need to ask your local butcher or deli to source it for you.

You can also substitute tuna or chicken for the ham.

Grate extra carrot and beetroot and store in the fridge for the next day's salad preparation.

Rainbow Tuna Salad

Tuna is full of protein and always a great back-up to have on hand. When creating dishes, aim to include as many colours of the rainbow as you can. It not only keeps it colourful (we eat with our eyes!) but it's a great way to ensure you are getting an array of nutrients.

SERVES 1

What's in it?

1 small can tuna (natural spring water or oil-based)

2 handfuls leafy greens

½ small carrot, grated

½ small yellow capsicum (pepper)

¼ cucumber

½ cup (1 small handful) finely sliced purple cabbage

Dressing

1 tbsp sesame oil

juice of ½ lemon

1 tbsp olive oil

sea salt and ground black pepper to taste

Place the leafy greens, grated carrot, capsicum, cucumber and purple cabbage in a bowl. Drain the tuna and add to the salad ingredients. In a small separate jar or bowl, shake or whisk the sesame oil, lemon, olive oil and salt and pepper together. Pour over the salad and gently combine. It doesn't get much simpler, right?

Tips

To save time, particularly if you like finely sliced vegetables, use a mandolin.

Always taste-test your dressings to get the perfect balance of flavours.

Baked Salmon and Green Salad

Fish is a great source of protein, so you're sure to get all the energy you need in your day as a super-busy mum when you indulge in this tasty dish. If you're a little reluctant to cook seafood, don't worry, this baked salmon dish is a no-fail recipe. We love how it stays super-moist and can be served cold the next day. Salmon is not only high in protein but also its good fats can reduce inflammation and improve heart health.

SERVES 1

What's in it?

150g fresh salmon fillet

1 tbsp olive oil

juice of ½ lemon

sea salt and ground pepper

Salad

2 small handfuls of lettuce
   or mixed salad leaves

6 cherry tomatoes, sliced

¼ cup (25g) black olives

Dressing

1–2 tbsp olive oil

1 tbsp lemon juice

sea salt and ground pepper

Preheat the oven to 170°C/325°F/gas 3. Rub the salmon with olive oil and lemon juice, and season with salt and pepper. Wrap the salmon in foil with the skin facing down.

Bake for 15–20 minutes until cooked through but not overcooked – the flesh should flake easily with a knife. Leave to stand in the foil for 3 minutes.

Meanwhile, put the lettuce in a bowl and add the tomatoes and olives. Put the dressing ingredients in a small bowl and whisk together. Add to the salad and toss to mix. Serve the salmon with the salad.

Tips

We love an extra squeeze of lemon juice on top of the salmon when serving.

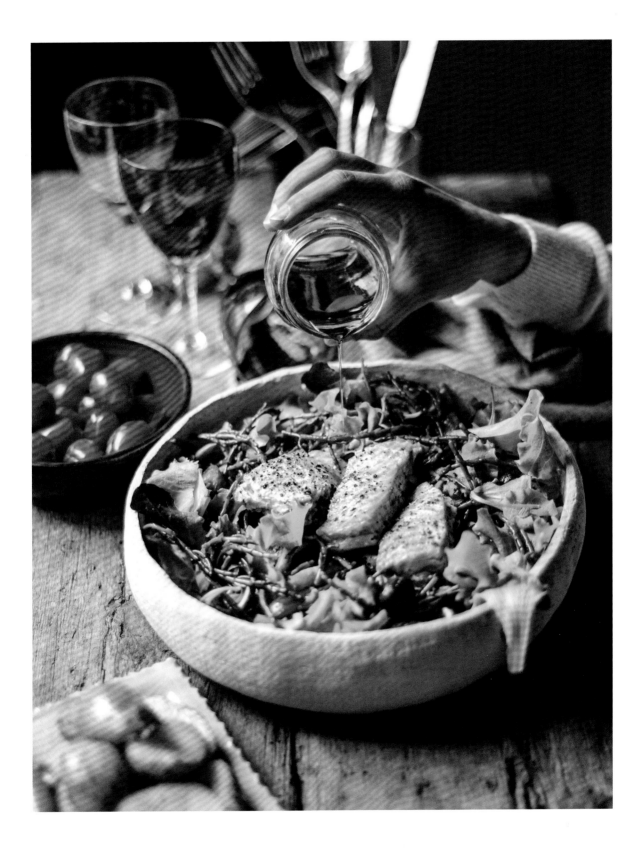

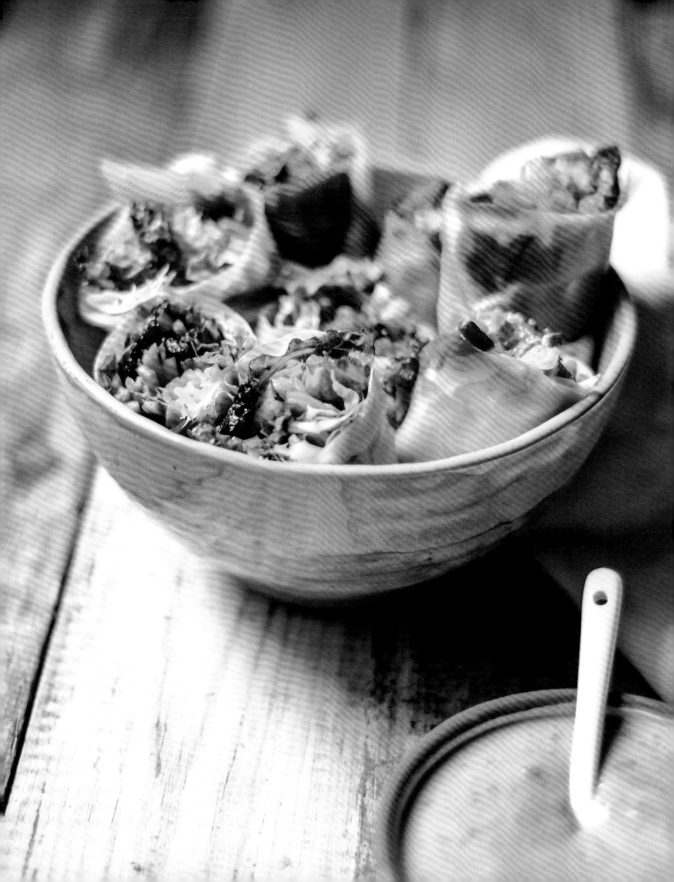

Rainbow Rice Paper Rolls

This dish is as tasty as it sounds colourful! Rainbow Rolls are a fun way to get extra vegetables into a meal and a great way to get the kids involved in the kitchen, by letting them choose their own fillings. If you want to add more protein, try including some leftover chicken, beef or a hard-boiled egg. The yogurt dressing can be used as a dipping sauce or sweetened with a little raw honey for fussy little eaters. We also love to add slices of fresh mango when available.

SERVES 1

What's in it?

1 carrot, finely sliced or grated

1 raw beetroot, finely sliced or grated

1 small handful of chopped loose lettuce leaves

½ mango

1 spring onion, thinly sliced

3 rice paper sheets

1 tbsp full-fat Greek or plain yogurt

1 tsp ground turmeric

Put the carrot, beetroot, lettuce, mango and spring onion in individual bowls. Pour warm water into a large bowl, then, one at a time, soak the rice paper sheets for 1 minute or until soft. Remove from the bowl and put on a slightly damp tea towel to drain off the excess water.

To make the yogurt dressing, put the yogurt in a small bowl and mix in the turmeric. Set aside.

Gently spread the yogurt dressing over each rice paper sheet. Layer the vegetables and mango down the middle of each sheet. Gently fold the bottom of the rice paper upwards, then fold in the two sides to hold all the ingredients together. Serve.

Tips

These rolls can be made the night before and are great for the kids' lunch boxes.

You can replace the rice paper with a wholemeal wrap, if you like.

Egg, Pear and Walnut Salad

Are you trying to find easier ways to get in your daily requirements of fruit? This salad has everything you'll need for a fresh fruit and veggie hit at lunchtime. Adding small amounts of fruit and nuts to your salads transforms them from boring and bland to tasty and satisfying. The added texture and crunch in this salad gets the juices flowing while adding extra nutrients and good fats. Don't be scared to experiment with this one: swap the eggs for chicken, the pear for apple and the walnuts for cashew nuts – whatever tickles your taste buds.

SERVES 1

What's in it?

2 medium eggs

2 handfuls assorted lettuce leaves

½ cup (1 small handful) finely sliced red cabbage

4 cherry tomatoes, quartered

½ spring onion, finely sliced

½ pear, finely sliced

½ cup (60g) walnuts

sea salt and ground black pepper

Dressing

1 tbsp full-fat Greek or plain yogurt

½ tsp curry powder

½ tsp honey (optional)

Cook the eggs in a saucepan of boiling water over a high heat for 4 minutes. Remove from the heat and gently peel off the shell. Put the lettuce in a bowl and add the cabbage, tomatoes, spring onion and pear. Mix together.

To make the dressing, put the yogurt in a small bowl and add the curry powder and honey, if using. Mix together until smooth and pour onto the salad. Stir through evenly. Cut the eggs in halves or quarters and put on top of the salad, then top with the walnuts.

Tips

Add chicken or bacon for extra protein.

Substitute apple for the pear.

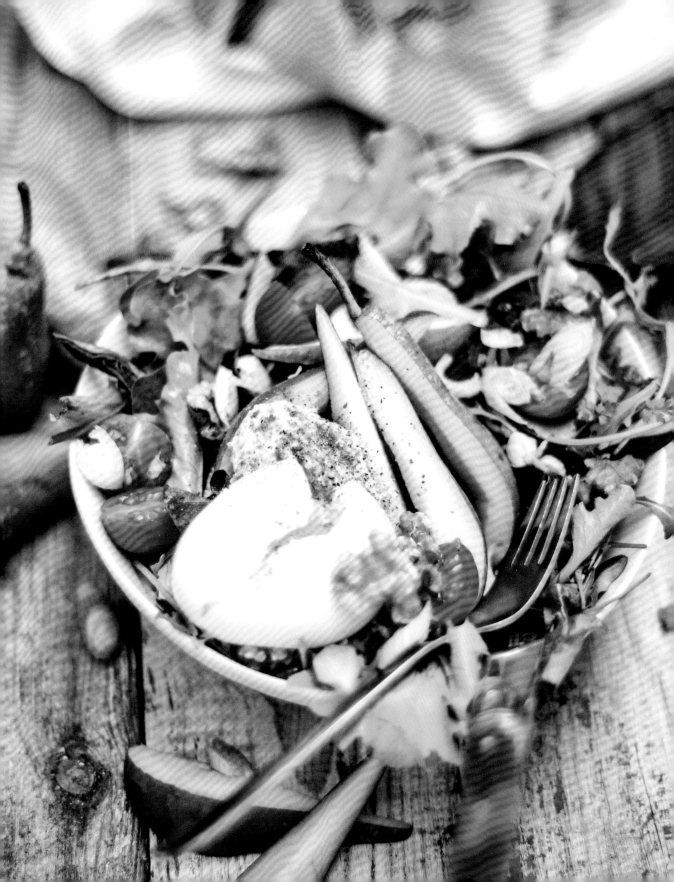

Soulful Mummy Platter

Having a little 'pick plate' for lunch is such a nutritious way to eat. It forces you to slow down and enjoy each bite.

What's in it?

1 small celery stalk, chopped into batons

½ small carrot, chopped into batons

5 cherry tomatoes

¼ cucumber, chopped into batons

1 boiled egg, halved

6 walnuts (or raw nuts of choice)

2 slices good-quality ham

Yogurt dip

3 tbsp natural yogurt

pinch of minced garlic

¼ cucumber, finely diced

Arrange the celery, carrot, cherry tomatoes, cucumber, eggs and walnuts in a circle around a small plate or platter. For the dressing, whisk the natural yogurt, minced garlic and cucumber together and place in a small dipping bowl. Place the bowl in the centre of the plate.

Tips

Make smaller versions for your kids and adapt to their age. It's a fun way to get them to try new raw foods.

You can substitute a yummy hummus for the yogurt dip.

Chicken, Spinach and Feta Patties

These tasty little babies are a family favourite and were the signature dish of Kimberley's late father. They are so simple, yet delish and great for the kids.

SERVES 4–5

What's in it?

500g lean chicken mince

250g frozen spinach, thawed and excess liquid drained

1½ cups (200g) crumbled feta (or goat's) cheese

1–2 tsp chilli paste

sea salt and ground black pepper to taste

Simply combine all the ingredients, roll the mixture into balls and flatten into patties. Gently fry for 3–4 minutes each side until cooked through and just golden. Serve with our staple green salad (see page 106)

Tips

Use turkey mince if chicken mince isn't available.

You can omit the chilli for the kids.

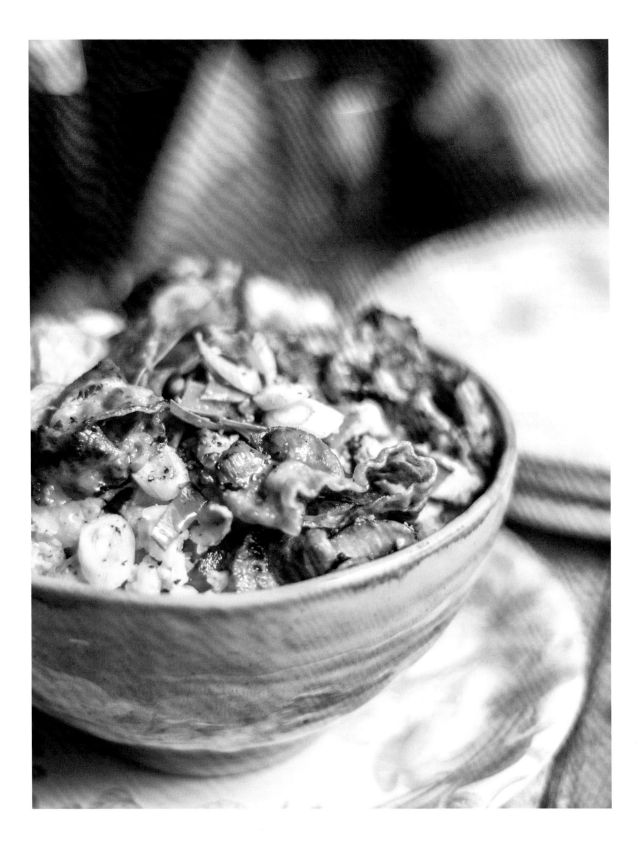

Bacon and Cauliflower Rice Bowl

Put a creative twist on your fried-rice dishes with this recipe. And we know your kids will enjoy it. This delight in a bowl is a much healthier version than fried rice. Cauliflower is lower in carbohydrates than rice and has a lovely nutty taste that complements the bacon and mushrooms. We like to make big batches at a time, so there are always leftovers for the next day.

SERVES 1

What's in it?

- 1 small cauliflower, cut into florets
- 2 tsp (10g) butter
- ¼ chopped onion
- ½ tsp crushed garlic
- 1 bacon rasher, finely chopped
- ½ cup (40g) sliced mushrooms
- 4 snow peas (mangetouts) finely sliced
- ½ spring onion, chopped, to garnish

Put the cauliflower in the food processor and blitz until it resembles rice. Heat the butter in a large frying pan over a medium heat and cook the onion, garlic, bacon and mushrooms until the bacon is crispy. Add the cauliflower rice to the frying pan and toss through for 1–2 minutes until all the ingredients are combined and the cauliflower rice is warmed though.

Remove from the heat and put in a bowl. Season with salt and pepper. Add the snow peas and garnish with spring onion.

Tips

This is the perfect side dish to serve with red meat, poultry or fish.

Mango and Coconut Sunshine Smoothie Bowl

On a hot summer's day, this mango and coconut smoothie bowl is a wonderful weekend lunch.

SERVES 1

What's in it?

½ cup (110g) frozen mango chunks

1 small frozen banana

½ cup (120ml) coconut milk

½ cup (120ml) coconut water

1 tsp raw honey

1 scoop natural protein powder

Place the frozen mango, banana, coconut milk, coconut water, protein and honey in a blender or food processor. Blitz until you get a thick, slushy texture. Pour into a bowl and top with sliced fruit, roasted nuts and toasted coconut flakes.

Tips

Depending on your blender or food processor, you may need to add more liquid, but the idea of a smoothie bowl is to ensure the contents stay thick.

Smoothie bowls are also delicious topped with gluten-free muesli.

Sticky Chicken Goodness Bowl

The raw crunch of the broccoli and apple in this bowl of goodness really sets off the salad. The sticky chicken provides the perfect protein component.

SERVES 1

What's in it?

2 handfuls leafy greens

3–4 broccoli florets, chopped

½ small apple, diced

½ small carrot, diced

handful of diced red capsicum (pepper)

¼ cucumber, diced

1 tbsp olive oil

1 tbsp apple cider vinegar

1 tsp pure honey

Protein topper

2 small chicken thigh fillets, diced

1 tsp coconut oil

2 tbsp tamari sauce

1 tbsp pure honey

generous sprinkle of garlic powder

Place all the salad vegetables in a bowl. Mix together the oil, vinegar and honey, pour the dressing over the vegetables, stir everything together and set aside.

Pan-fry the thigh pieces in coconut oil for 5–7 minutes. When almost cooked through, pour in the tamari, honey and garlic powder and quickly toss so as not to burn. Cover and let it rest for 5 minutes. Serve on top of the salad.

Tips

For extra flavour and tenderness, marinate the chicken in the tamari sauce overnight. Make up a few extra batches and place in wraps for the kids' lunch boxes.

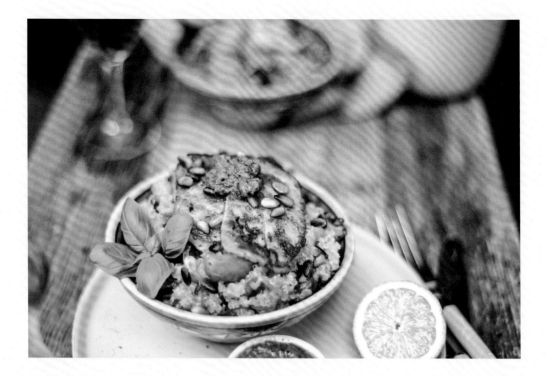

Delightful dinners

Too often, traditional family dinners get lost in the duties of parenting. Parents become exhausted and time-poor, and family meals become less of a social event and more something to get out of the way. Having family meals together, however, can enhance family dynamics and foster positive family relationships. And meals don't have to be difficult to prepare or expensive to put on the table.

Often, dinner is the only time when all the family members can manage to be present at the table at one time. This section is filled with delicious healthy dinner recipes that the whole family can enjoy. We would urge you, however, that although the following recipes are yummo, it's important to note that when we are trying to lose weight we shouldn't overeat, particularly later in the evenings, when our bodies won't have a chance to work off the extra calories. Keeping portion sizes in check will be an important part of helping you reach your health-and-fitness goals.

Bacon and Mushroom Frittata

Frittatas make for fantastic family meals. You'll need just a little time to whip this one up, and the family will be singing your praises yet again. What a way to celebrate with family – over an easy, nutritious, yet simple, meal. This frittata has made it into our hearts for a no-stress but nutritious midweek meal. Simply serve with a fresh salad from our recipe list for a complete meal.

SERVES 4

What's in it?

- 1 tbsp olive oil, plus extra for greasing
- 4–5 bacon rashers (no added nitrates), chopped
- 6 button mushrooms, sliced
- 2 spring onions, finely sliced
- 10 medium eggs at room temperature
- ½ cup (125ml) almond milk, or your milk of choice
- ½ cup (60g) crumbled goat's cheese
- sea salt and ground black pepper

Preheat the oven to 180°C/350°F/gas 4. Line a baking tin with baking paper, then grease the paper. Heat the oil in a small frying pan over a medium heat and add the bacon and mushrooms. Cook for 5 minutes or until the bacon is crispy, then stir in the spring onions. Spread the bacon, mushrooms and spring onions evenly over the prepared baking tin.

Whisk the eggs and milk together and season with salt and pepper. Pour the mixture into the baking tin, covering the mushroom mixture. Sprinkle the goat's cheese evenly on top.

Bake for 20–30 minutes until cooked through. Serve.

Tips

Be careful not to over-bake the frittata.

You can also have this for breakfast or as a snack, and leftovers can be frozen.

Spiced Lamb with Baked Veggies and Feta

Here's a meat-lover's favourite. It's old school with a load of spice and punch, and we're sure it will become a new weekend favourite and another reason why your family and friends will come to visit. Baked vegetables are comfort food at its best. The baking enhances the flavours, bringing out their natural sweetness, which the kids love. We love to use minced lamb and rosemary here, but you can easily replace it with beef or chicken and use different herbs, if you like.

SERVES 4

What's in it?

1 large sweet potato, cut into small cubes

2 medium beetroot, cut into small cubes

1 red onion, cut into chunks

1 tbsp coconut oil, melted

leaves from 3 rosemary sprigs

500g minced lamb

1 pinch of dried chilli flakes

1 tsp olive oil, if needed

4 handfuls spinach or other dark leafy greens

1 cup (170g) cherry tomatoes, sliced

¼ cup (30g) cubed feta cheese

1 avocado, pitted, skinned and cubed

sea salt and ground black pepper

Dressing

1 tbsp olive oil

2 tsp lemon juice

1 garlic clove, crushed

Preheat the oven to 180°C/350°F/gas 4 and line a baking tray with baking paper. Put the sweet potato, beetroot and onion in a large bowl and add the oil and half the rosemary, then toss together to coat. Lay the vegetables evenly over the prepared baking tray and then season with salt and pepper. Bake for 30 minutes or until the sweet potato and beetroot are soft on the inside and crispy on the outside.

Meanwhile, heat a frying pan over a medium heat and add the lamb, chilli flakes and the leftover rosemary. Season with salt and pepper. You may need to add a little water or olive oil if the mince starts to dry out. Cook the mince until brown.

Put all the dressing ingredients into a small bowl and whisk to combine. Season with salt and pepper.

To serve, layer each plate with spinach, cherry tomatoes and baked vegetables. Top with the lamb mince, then crumble the feta over the top, finish with the avocado and drizzle with the dressing.

Tips

Leftovers can be stored in the fridge for lunch the next day.

Replace the feta with goat's cheese, if you prefer.

Minced lamb can be replaced with beef, chicken or turkey.

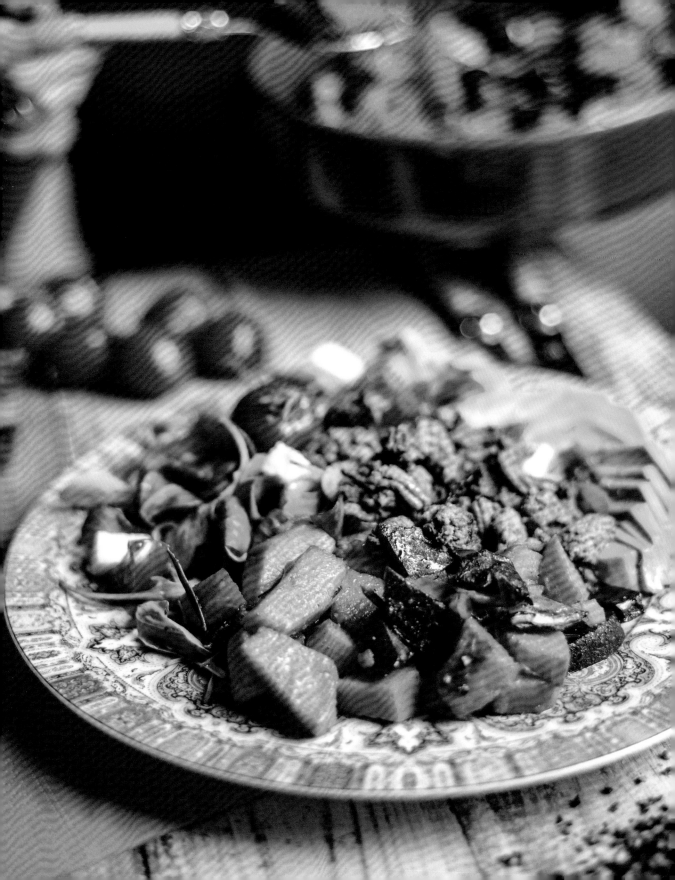

Lamb Shank and Vegetable Soup

Hearty soups are great fillers and an easy back-up to have to hand. They freeze well and can be jam-packed with vegetables. This recipe will not disappoint when it comes to flavour either. The lamb shanks take a while to cook but they bring an extra heartiness to the recipe. Keep in mind that they can be replaced with sweet potato or quinoa for a vegetarian version.

SERVES 6–8

What's in it?

- 1 tbsp olive oil
- 1 leek, sliced
- 2 onions, finely chopped
- 2 garlic cloves, crushed
- ½ head of cauliflower, cut into florets
- 1 head of broccoli, cut into florets
- 2 zucchini (courgettes), chopped
- 2 capsicums (peppers), any colour, deseeded and sliced
- 2 lamb shanks, excess fat removed
- 8 cups (2 litres) water
- 400g can chopped tomatoes (no salt or sugar added)
- sea salt and ground black pepper

Using a very large saucepan, heat the olive oil over a medium heat and add the leek, onions and garlic, then cook for 5 minutes or until soft. Add the cauliflower, broccoli, zucchini and capsicums. Add the lamb shanks, water and tomatoes. Give the mixture a good stir. The lamb shanks should be almost covered with water.

Put the lid on the pan and bring to the boil, then reduce the heat and simmer for at least 2 hours or until the lamb falls off the bone. Stir often and check that the water level doesn't get too low. Remove the pan from the heat and carefully remove the lamb shanks – they will be hot. Remove the meat from the bone and shred it with a fork. Set the meat aside.

Using a hand-held stick blender, purée the soup until smooth. Add the lamb and stir through. Season with salt and pepper. Serve.

Tips

For extra flavour, you can use home-made stock instead of water (see Bone Broth on page 151).

Any leftovers won't go to waste, as you can freeze it for last-minute meals.

This dish can be made in a slow cooker to save time and energy. It will take about 6 hours.

Beef Stir-Fry

A stir-fry is quick and easy to prepare and it's quick to cook too, making it a speciality in our kitchens. Gone are the days when we reached for the highly processed packet stir-fry sauce. With fresh ingredients and a little seasoning, this healthy stir-fry is simple. Spice it up by adding a fresh chilli for extra punch. We like to double the ingredients so that we have lunch ready for the next day.

SERVES 4

What's in it?

- 1 tbsp coconut oil, plus extra if needed
- 500g frying beef, cut into strips
- 1 garlic clove, crushed
- 1 thumb-sized piece of root ginger, peeled and grated
- 4 spring onions, chopped
- 1 cup (140g) green beans cut into 2.5cm pieces
- 1 cup (75g) sliced capsicum (pepper)
- 1 cup (70g) sliced button mushrooms
- 3–4 tbsp tamari (wheat-free soy sauce)
- 1/3 cup (80ml) water
- 1 tbsp raw honey
- 1 tsp arrowroot (gluten-free thickener)

Heat the coconut oil in a frying pan over a medium-high heat and add the beef strips. Cook until it is no longer pink then remove from pan. Add a little more coconut oil if needed, reduce the heat to medium and fry the garlic, ginger, onion and remaining vegetables. Cook for about 5 minutes.

In a small bowl, whisk together the tamari, water, honey and arrowroot. Return the beef strips to the pan of vegetables and stir in the sauce. Heat through, being careful not to overcook. Serve.

Tips

Serve with brown rice, zucchini (courgette) noodles or quinoa.

Leftovers make the best ready-made lunch.

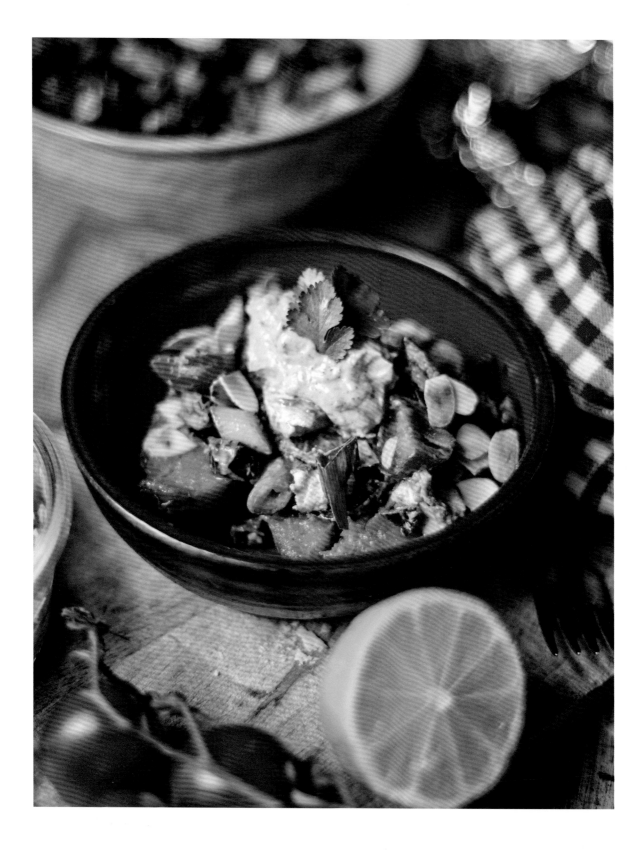

Stuffed Sweet Potato with Chicken and Creamy Avocado Dressing

This stuffed potato dish has a light freshness that is super-tasty. We like to use barbecued or poached chicken that has been made in advance, then it is simply mixed with the red cabbage salad and the creamy dressing. We love to squeeze extra lime on top.

SERVES 4

What's in it?

- 4 medium sweet potatoes, unpeeled
- 4 cups (240g) finely sliced red cabbage
- 4 spring onions, sliced
- 2 cups (340g) cherry tomatoes, quartered
- 4 cups (600g) cooked shredded chicken
- ¼ cup (20g) toasted slivered (flaked) almonds

Dressing

- 1 avocado, pitted, skinned and roughly chopped
- 1 garlic clove
- ½ tbsp lime juice
- ¼ cup (60ml) olive oil or Greek yogurt
- ¼ cup (4 tbsp) cilantro (coriander)
- 1 tsp sea salt and ground black pepper

To make the dressing, put all the ingredients into a blender or food processor. Blend together until creamy smooth. Set aside or store in a container in the fridge.

Preheat the oven to 170°C/325°F/gas 3. Wrap the sweet potatoes in foil, then put them on a baking tray and bake for 40 minutes or until they are soft in the middle; test by pricking them with a knife or fork.

Meanwhile, put the cabbage in a large bowl and add the spring onions, tomatoes and chicken. Pour in half the avocado dressing and stir through, covering all the vegetables.

When the potatoes are soft inside, remove the foil and slice down the middle but not all the way through. Make a hole in the middle and add the chicken mixture. Top with toasted almonds and drizzle the remaining avocado dressing over the top. Serve.

Tips

Use the leftover red cabbage salad for lunch the next day.

The creamy avocado dressing can be stored in the fridge for up to 1 week. We love to dip our raw vegetables in it for a healthy snack.

Sweet Potato Curry with Prawns

Yup, another sweet potato recipe (we told you we love 'em). Curry is a family favourite of ours. It's full of flavour, and this simple recipe is light and tasty. Coconut cream can be replaced with Greek yogurt for a lighter version if you like. Serve with brown rice or quinoa.

SERVES 4

What's in it?

1 tbsp coconut oil

2 onions, finely chopped

1–2 garlic cloves, to taste, crushed

2 tsp cumin seeds

2 tsp mustard seeds

3 tbsp curry powder

2 x 400g cans chopped tomatoes

2 large sweet potatoes, peeled and cut into cubes

2 cups (500ml) vegetable stock

4 cups (4 large handfuls) mixed vegetables, such as cauliflower, zucchini (courgette), carrot

12 king prawns, peeled

½ cup (100g) coconut cream or full-fat Greek yogurt

Heat the coconut oil in a large, deep frying pan over a medium heat and add the onions, garlic and spices. Cook for 5 minutes or until fragrant and the onion is translucent.

Add the tomatoes, potatoes and stock to the pan. Bring to the boil, then add the remaining vegetables. Simmer for about 10–15 minutes or until the sweet potato is tender. Add the prawns and simmer for 5 minutes or until cooked through. Stir in the coconut cream. Serve.

Tips

Add a little extra coconut cream on top and garnish with fresh herbs, if you like.

Be careful not to over-cook the prawns.

Almond-Coated Chicken with Red Cabbage Coleslaw

This one sounds a little fancy, doesn't it? But although it might sound like a restaurant meal, you really can whip it up yourself. And when you do, we know that the praise will flow. This take on the traditional chicken schnitzel is much healthier and tastier too. Almond meal (ground almonds) is a gluten-free alternative to breadcrumbs, and the flavour is complemented when cooked in coconut oil, which is ideal for frying at a high temperature.

SERVES 4

What's in it?

1½ cups (150g) almond meal (ground almonds)

1 tbsp dried mixed herbs

12 chicken tenderloins or 4 chicken breasts, cut into strips

1–2 tbsp coconut oil, as needed

½ small red cabbage, finely sliced or shredded

4 spring onions, finely sliced

2 celery sticks, finely sliced

¼ cup (20g) toasted slivered (flaked) almonds

sea salt and ground black pepper

Dressing

⅓ cup (75g) tahini

⅓ cup (80ml) water

juice of ½ lemon

1 garlic clove, crushed

1–2 tsp raw honey, to taste

Preheat the oven to 180°C/350°F/gas 4 and line a baking tray with baking paper. Put the almond meal in a bowl and season with salt, pepper and the herbs. Pour the almond meal onto a large plate. Coat the individual chicken tenderloins in the almond mixture and press down firmly. Set aside.

Heat the coconut oil in a large frying pan over a medium heat and gently brown the almond-coated chicken for a few minutes on each side. Remove them from the frying pan and put them on the prepared baking tray. Bake for 10 minutes or until cooked through.

Meanwhile, put the dressing ingredients in a small bowl and whisk together well. Season with salt and pepper.

Put the cabbage in a large bowl and add the spring onions and celery. Toss the dressing through the salad until completely covered. Garnish with the toasted almonds. Serve the salad with the chicken.

Tips

Add extra water to the dressing if you prefer a runnier consistency.

Leftovers store well in the fridge for lunch the next day.

You can use natural almond or peanut butter instead of tahini.

Warm Quinoa and Halloumi Salad with Pesto

This dish is so easy to love. With a really fresh, vibrant and healthy balance, we think this may become a regular at your dinner table. Quinoa is the perfect gluten-free alternative for sensitive tummies. It is technically a seed and is high in protein and has a subtle nutty taste and texture similar to barley or buckwheat. It's important to wash it thoroughly before cooking to remove its natural coating and bitterness. We always have a pre-made batch in the fridge ready to bulk up any meal.

SERVES 4

What's in it?

- 2 zucchini (courgettes), cut in 1cm thick pieces
- 1 red capsicum (pepper), cut into squares
- 1 yellow or green capsicum (pepper), cut into squares
- 1 red onion, sliced
- 4 Roma (plum) tomatoes, quartered
- 1 tbsp and 1 tsp olive oil
- 2 cups (340g) quinoa
- 12 fine slices of halloumi
- ½ cup (30g) toasted pine nuts
- salt and ground black pepper

Pesto

- 2 cups (50g) basil leaves
- 2 garlic cloves
- ¾ cup (45g) roasted pine nuts
- ⅓ cup (80ml) olive oil
- juice of ½ small lemon
- 1 tsp sea salt

Preheat the oven to 170°C/325°F/gas 3 and line a large baking tray with baking paper.

Put the zucchini in a large bowl and add the peppers, onion and tomatoes, then add 1 tbsp olive oil. Mix through, making sure the vegetables are covered with oil. Season with salt and pepper, then lay the vegetables in the prepared baking tray. Bake for 30 minutes or until the vegetables are soft – be careful not to burn them.

Rinse the quinoa thoroughly in a small sieve under running water, rubbing the quinoa with your hands. Put it into a pan with 4 cups (1 litre) of water over a high heat. When the water is boiling, reduce the heat and simmer for 15 minutes or until the water is absorbed and the quinoa seeds start to 'sprout'. Turn off the heat and put the lid on for 10 minutes or until the quinoa has fully absorbed the liquid. Fluff the quinoa with a fork and set aside with the lid on to keep warm.

Meanwhile, to make the pesto, put all the ingredients into a food processor and blitz them until smooth. Tip into a small bowl or container and set aside.

In a small frying pan heat 1 tsp olive oil over a medium heat. Fry the halloumi a few minutes on each side or until golden.

We like to serve this dish layered on a large serving platter with the quinoa as a base, then the vegetables and topped with halloumi. Drizzle with the pesto sauce and top with the pine nuts. Or simply divide into individual bowls.

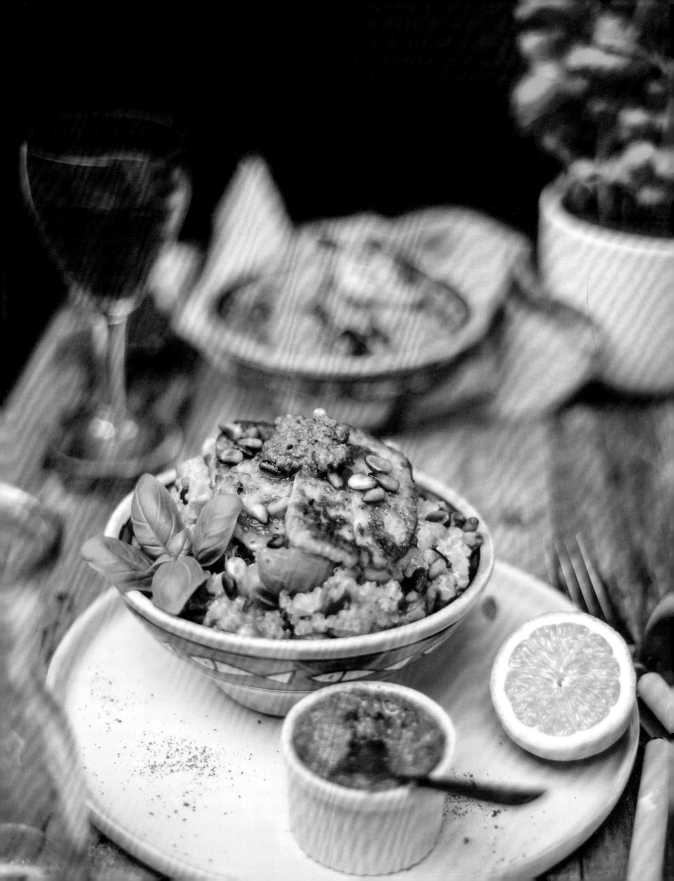

Spiced Barbecue Steak and Jacket Potato

This sizzling meal will leave your family and guests wanting more. Its simplicity means that it's really easy to make, yet it should hit the spot with every family member. The humble baked potato is a perfect accompaniment to this dish and although it gets a bad rap when it comes to fat loss, it is a wholefood that is high in fibre and is fine if eaten in moderate portions.

SERVES 4

What's in it?

4 small potatoes, unpeeled and skins washed

800g beef rump steak

1 tbsp olive oil

1 tbsp Moroccan spice or similar

4 tbsp full-fat sour cream

salt and ground black pepper

Salad

4 handfuls of mixed lettuce or salad leaves, such as rocket and baby spinach

3 Roma (plum) tomatoes, quartered

1 cucumber, sliced

1 avocado, pitted, peeled and sliced

½ red onion, sliced

Dressing

1 tbsp extra virgin olive oil

juice of ½ lemon

Preheat the oven to 180°C/350°F/gas 4. Wrap the potatoes individually in foil. Bake for 30–40 minutes until soft inside when squeezed. The amount of time to cook will vary, depending on the size of the potato.

Meanwhile, rub the steaks with olive oil and sprinkle with spice and salt and pepper on both sides, making sure that they are generously covered. Preheat your barbecue to a high temperature, or preheat a grill or large, heavy frying pan to medium-high. Put the steaks on the barbecue (or add the steaks to the grill pan or frying pan). Cook for 4–5 minutes on each side. Remove and leave the steaks on a plate to rest for 5 minutes before serving.

While the steak is resting, put the salad ingredients in a large bowl. Drizzle with olive oil and squeeze over the lemon juice, then season with salt and pepper. Gently give the salad a toss so that it's evenly coated with the dressing.

Take the potatoes out of the oven and remove the foil. Slice them down the middle and top with a dollop of sour cream. Serve the steak with the potatoes and salad.

Tips

We like to cut the steak finely into strips before serving.

Caramelised Onion Pizza

Pizza is always a hit with the kids. Deciding which ingredients will be healthy enough to cover your pizza base with is not always easy, though, so we've taken the worry out of it for you with this deliciously crafty home-made pizza recipe. If you're looking for a healthier Friday night indulgence, this pizza hits the spot. Caramelised onions are traditionally cooked for a long period of time, but ours are quick and, we think, super-tasty, and they blend perfectly with the sweet potato, goat's cheese and pine nuts.

SERVES 4

What's in it?

1 sweet potato, finely sliced

1 tbsp coconut oil, melted

1 tbsp butter

3 red onions, sliced

4 medium-small wholemeal pitta breads (gluten-free if possible)

1 cup (200g) pizza base tomato sauce

1 small handful of spinach

½ cup (25g) fresh basil leaves, chopped

1 avocado, pitted, skinned and sliced

½ cup (60g) crumbled goat's cheese or feta

¼ cup (30g) toasted pine nuts

Preheat the oven to 170°C/325°F/gas 3 and line a large baking tray with baking paper. Put the sweet potato in a large bowl and add the oil. Mix well to coat thoroughly, then lay the sweet potato in the prepared baking tray. Bake for 10–15 minutes until crisp.

Meanwhile, heat the butter in a small frying pan over a medium heat and cook the onions for 10–15 minutes until they soften and start to caramelise to a dark brown colour.

Spread the pitta breads evenly with pizza tomato sauce. When the sweet potato is cooked, remove it from the oven and lay flat on top of the sauce, then spread the caramelised onion and spinach evenly over each. Transfer to a pizza tray or baking sheet and bake for 10 minutes or until the base is warmed through. Remove from the oven and top with basil, avocado, goat's cheese and toasted pine nuts.

Tips

Keep an eye on these while they are in the oven, as they can cook quickly.

The recipe is for four people, but it can be adapted to just one person, or for more!

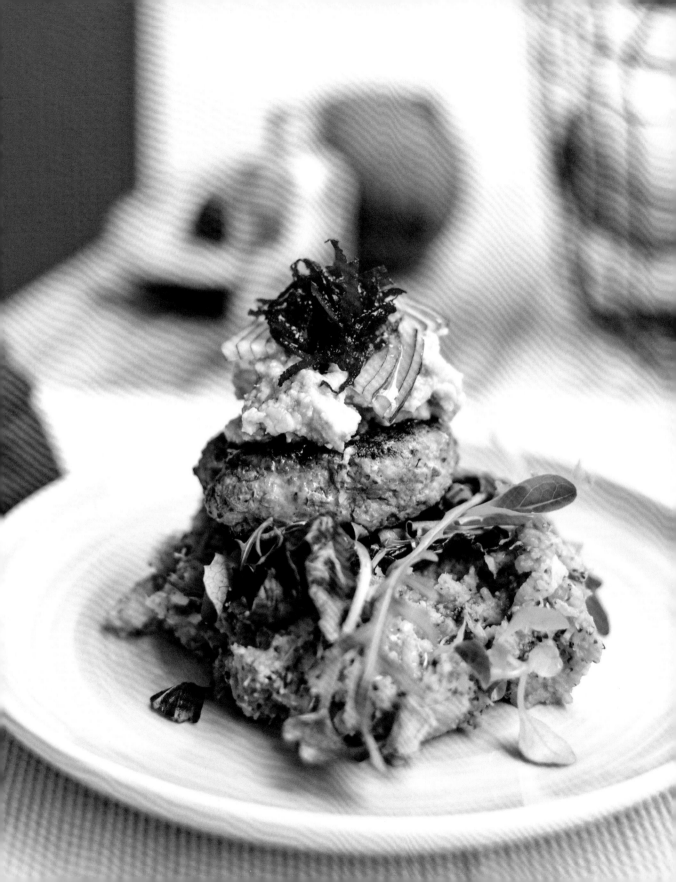

Gourmet Meat Patties

If you want the perfect way to spice up a burger for the family and watch the kilos at the same time, we have the answer here. It's a simple uptake of the beloved hamburger by replacing the bun with mashed vegetables. This is a great way to add nutritional value to a meal without compromising taste. The crunch of the salad and creaminess of the avocado topping has made this a dinnertime favourite of ours.

SERVES 4

What's in it?

500g minced beef

1 egg, beaten

1 garlic clove, crushed

1 tsp Dijon mustard

½ cup (40g) grated zucchini (courgette)

1 tsp sea salt

½ tsp ground black pepper

Mash

1 sweet potato, peeled and diced

2 cups (120g) broccoli florets

1 tbsp butter

Salad

1 avocado, pitted and skinned

2 tbsp goat's cheese

1 tsp butter

1 red onion, sliced

2 handfuls mixed lettuce leaves

½ cup (60g) grated raw beetroot

1 tsp sea salt

½ tsp ground black pepper

In a large bowl combine the beef, egg, garlic, mustard, zucchini, salt and pepper. With clean, slightly wet hands, shape the mixture into four evenly sized burgers. Set aside in the fridge until ready to cook.

Cook the patties on a barbecue or in a frying pan, in a little oil, over a medium heat for 12–15 minutes, turning halfway through. When cooked to your liking, remove and set aside. Cover with foil to keep warm.

Meanwhile, boil or steam the sweet potato and broccoli until it is soft. Heat the 1 tsp butter in a small frying pan over a medium heat and cook the onion until soft, then remove and set aside. Put the sweet potato and broccoli in a bowl then add the 1 tbsp butter and mash together with a fork or potato masher.

Put the avocado and goat's cheese in a small bowl and mash together until creamy. Put the patties on individual plates and layer with the mash and salad, finishing with the avocado and goat's cheese topper. Enjoy!

Chicken and Turmeric Casserole

If you're not familiar with turmeric, you're missing out, because it has a great flavour and is also very good for you. Try this mouth-watering, tasty meal and your whole family will rave about your culinary skills. Casseroles are a mum's best friend because they can be made in advance with minimal fuss, and any leftovers always taste even better the next day. This sweet-tasting recipe contains turmeric and ginger – magical spices that have immune-boosting properties. The casserole is naturally sweetened with dates – and the kids will love it too.

SERVES 6

What's in it?

- 2 large red onions, roughly chopped
- 2 thumbnail-sized pieces of raw turmeric, peeled
- 2–3 thumbnail-sized pieces of root ginger, peeled
- 1 small red chilli, deseeded (optional)
- 2 garlic cloves
- 1 tbsp coconut oil
- 1kg chicken breasts, cubed
- 400ml can coconut milk
- 1 tbsp vegetable bouillon powder dissolved in 1 cup (250ml) hot water
- 4–5 dried pitted dates, to taste, chopped
- 4 large handfuls of kale or leafy greens
- 1 large handful of fresh basil leaves

Preheat the oven to 180°C/350°F/gas 4. Put the onions in a food processor and add the turmeric, ginger, chilli and garlic. Blitz until you get a chunky paste.

Heat the coconut oil in a flameproof casserole or frying pan over a medium heat and cook the paste until the onion is translucent and the spices are fragrant.

Add the chicken and cook until browned, then add the coconut milk and stock. Stir and cook for 10 minutes. If using a frying pan, transfer to a casserole.

Cover the casserole and put in the oven for 45 minutes–1 hour, stirring occasionally, then stir in the dates, kale and basil. Cook in the oven for another 15 minutes, then serve.

Tips

Remember to stir the casserole a few times.

Serve the dish on its own or with brown rice, zucchini (courgette) noodles or quinoa.

You can also make this dish with lamb or beef but you will need to cook it for longer.

Mexican Mince Lettuce Cups

Have you always wanted to be able to whip up a great Mexican dish but you didn't know which one to try? This meal will bring out the *arriba!* in you and your little ones. It's a true touch of Mexico without the hassle or cost. This is one of those fun meals that everyone loves; we have simply replaced the traditional taco shell with lettuce to make a healthier version. If the kids aren't convinced, replace the lettuce wrap with a wholemeal pitta bread or wrap.

SERVES 4

What's in it?

1 tbsp olive oil

1 onion, finely chopped

1 garlic clove, crushed

6 mushrooms, sliced

500g lean minced beef

400g can tomatoes (no added salt or sugar)

2 tsp taco seasoning or Mexican spice (no salt or sugar)

dried chilli flakes (optional)

10–12 cos lettuce leaves to use as 'cups'

½ red, yellow and green capsicum (pepper), deseeded and sliced into thin strips

2 spring onions, finely sliced

½ cup (100g) full-fat sour cream

Heat the olive oil in a large frying pan over a medium heat and add the onion, garlic and mushrooms. Cook for 5 minutes or until the onions are translucent. Add the beef to the frying pan and cook until brown, then add the tomatoes and spices.

Cover the frying pan, reduce the heat and simmer for 20 minutes, stirring occasionally. Remove the mince from the frying pan and tip into a large bowl. Divide the mince among each lettuce cup and top with capsicum, spring onion and ½ tsp sour cream for each. Serve.

Tips

Season the mince with chilli flakes when cooking, if you like a little extra heat.

Instead of making individual servings, you can put all the ingredients in separate bowls and everyone can serve themselves.

Chicken and Zucchini Noodles with Creamy Basil Sauce

This one has to be on our favourite of all the favourites lists! We're replacing flour products with tasty, fresh zucchini. It's super-healthy and super-tasty – for super-busy mums. Zucchini noodles are the perfect gluten-free replacement for traditional pasta; the gluten in pasta can leave you bloated and it can also hamper fat loss.

SERVES 4

What's in it?

5 zucchini (courgettes)

½ tbsp and 2 tsp coconut oil

12 chicken tenderloins or 4 chicken breasts, cut into strips

1 tbsp almond meal (ground almonds)

1 tbsp pine nuts

basil leaves and toasted pine nuts, to garnish

Basil sauce

2 cups (240g) raw cashew nuts (soaked in water for 4 hours or until softened)

6 large fresh basil leaves

¾ cup (200ml) water, plus extra if needed

2 tbsp olive oil

juice of ½ lemon

1 garlic clove

1–2 tsp Bragg's seasoning or a dash of tamari (wheat-free soy sauce)

1 tsp sea salt, or to taste

In advance, blend the basil sauce ingredients in a blender or food processor until the sauce is silky smooth. You may need to add more water to get the desired consistency, but it shouldn't be so runny that it falls off a spoon. Check and adjust the seasoning.

Using a vegetable peeler, slice the zucchini into ribbons. Set aside. Heat ½ tbsp coconut oil in a large frying pan over a medium-high heat and add the chicken. Cook for 2–3 minutes each side, then reduce the heat, cover and cook for 2–3 minutes until the chicken is cooked through. Meanwhile, put 2 tsp oil in a separate frying pan over a medium heat and add the almond meal and pine nuts. Toast until golden – this should only take about 3 minutes. Add the zucchini noodles and toss with the almond mixture until coated and warmed through.

Put the noodles on a platter, layer with the chicken and top with basil sauce. Garnish with extra basil leaves and toasted pine nuts.

Tips

We like to make the zucchini noodles and basil dressing in advance so that it's just a matter of toasting the almond meal and cooking the chicken on the day.

The creamy sauce is dairy-free, and it can be stored in the fridge and used as a tasty dip or complement to any meat dish.

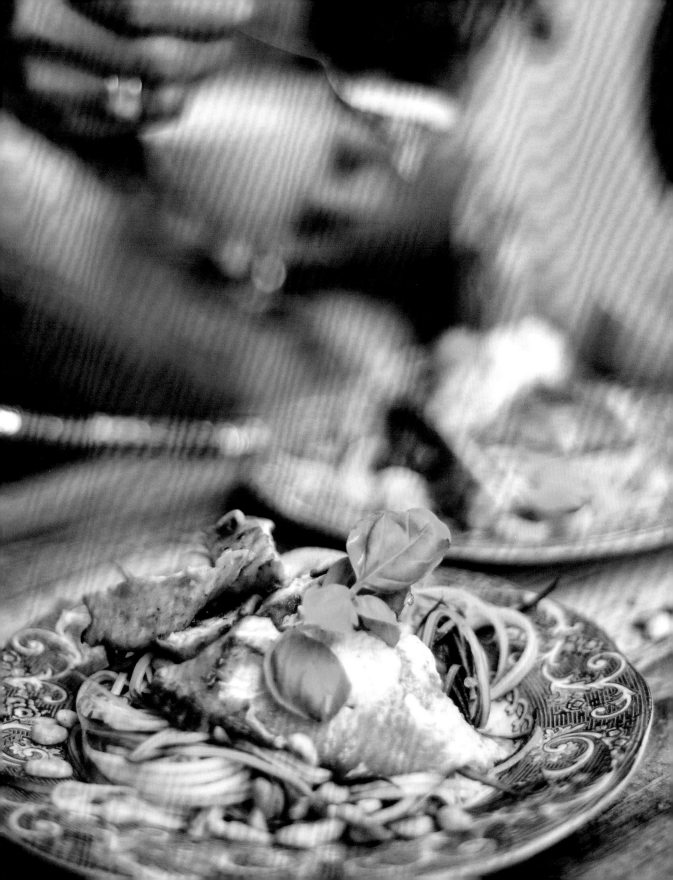

Healthy sweet treats

Sweets! Okay, we have your attention now, don't we? The healthy sweet treats in this section are not included in the four-week Stay Strong Mummy Plan, but they will make an irresistible special something, and we know you'll fall in love with them as much as we have.

We all enjoy a small indulgence every now and then, so it's important to make sure that we have healthy options available for when the need arises. A sweet treat is exactly that: it's a treat! Don't over-eat these yummy delights – we've done it ourselves and quickly learned that it's an easy way to sabotage fat-loss goals.

Our bodies are simply not designed to process large amounts of sugar, even the healthier natural versions like honey, maple syrup, and even fruit, so although they are delightful, if you want to look and feel your best and keep the guilt at bay, keep these treats to a minimum.

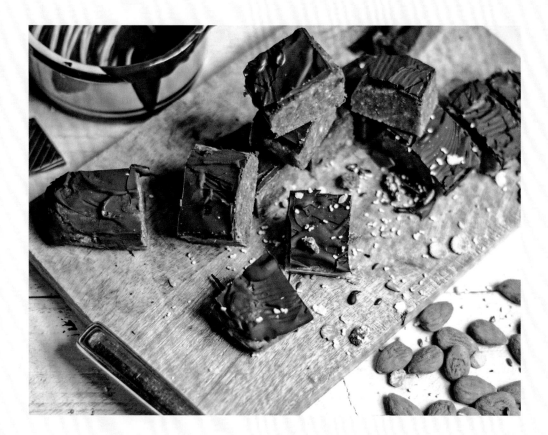

Treat meals – no guilt necessary

The old 'cheat' meal has been around for decades. A lot of mainstream diets out there recommend their followers have a cheat day, which often sees people spiralling out of control and bingeing on sugar and other processed foods, leaving themselves feeling fuzzy, slow and lethargic by the Monday morning. We aren't fans of the word 'cheat' or the craze of a 'cheat day' – here's why. We both believe in having a balanced approach to living a healthy, energetic and happy life. Not just for us, but for our families. It's quite hard for a lot of people to find that balance between eating and exercising well, and enjoying a night in the living room with the family indulging in a pizza. And that's generally because they feel so restricted when it comes to mainstream diets. It's also usually because they have deprived their body of one of the macronutrients (protein, fat, carb) and when their body has a taste of it, it's like a switch is flicked and they simply cannot stop eating. That few slices of pizza turns into a whole pizza, a tub of ice-cream and some biscuits for good measure.

When you find your flow with clean eating, you'll soon notice that you can enjoy a treat meal once a week, without having that 'emotional' switch flicking. Here's our take on it: first of all, notice that we said 'treat' meal and not 'cheat' meal. We don't believe that you associate the word 'cheat' with a meal, because you're not cheating. We believe that it's important for your body to be able to process small amounts of processed foods. Yeah, sure, ideally it would be great if we could live 100 per cent clean and organic, but for two busy mums (with toddlers and teens), the reality is that we haven't chosen that path. Our kids enjoy a piece of cake at a birthday party, we love a pizza and wine with our husbands, our kids love an ice-cream outing with their grandparents and we love our hot chips!

On our programme (and beyond), you are allowed a treat meal once a week. And you are told to *enjoy* it! Lose any negative stigma. When you take this approach, you'll notice that you start to lose that all-or-nothing approach to your health. You'll notice that your energy levels might slump a little soon after the meal and (while it's not our favourite feeling in the world) it's actually good for you to acknowledge how the processed foods makes you feel after eating them. It'll slide, as it's only one meal (not an entire day), and you'll be even more determined and motivated to indulge in that protein smoothie once again.

Strawberry Chia Pudding

We know how tricky it can be to avoid sweet treats when you're watching your weight or trying to help your family to eat healthily, but it's time to celebrate as you devour these perfectly healthy and super-tasty treats with a difference. Chia seeds are a well-known superfood that has become very popular. They are high in omega-3 fatty acids and protein, and they are great for your digestion. It's important to soak them to get the full benefit of the nutrients. The seeds are flavourless and they swell to up to 12 times their original size, creating a gelatine-type consistency. We love to soak our chia seeds in almond milk, and then add berries to make a sweet snack that everyone loves.

SERVES 1

What's in it?

1 heaped tbsp chia seeds

½ cup (125ml) almond milk or coconut milk

1 cup (100g) strawberries, sliced

4 fresh mint leaves, chopped

1 tsp honey

Put the chia seeds in a small serving bowl and add the almond milk. Leave for 5 minutes or until soaked and expanded.

Layer the strawberries on top of the chia seeds. Top with mint and honey for extra sweetness.

Tips

Make sure you give the chia seeds a good stir when soaking in the almond milk.

Choose other fruit in season if strawberries are not available.

Frozen berries are also great to use if you don't have fresh strawberries.

This can be made the night before for an easy on-the-go snack.

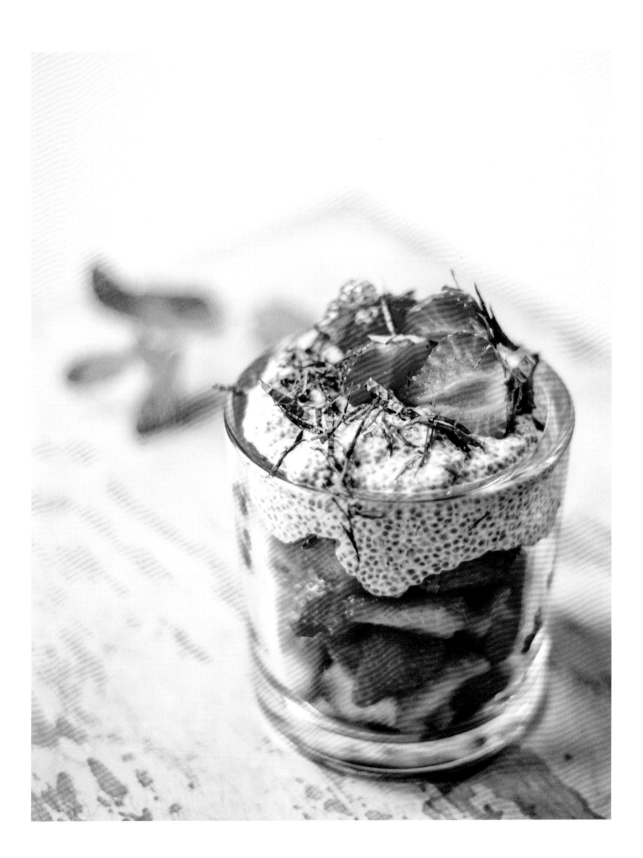

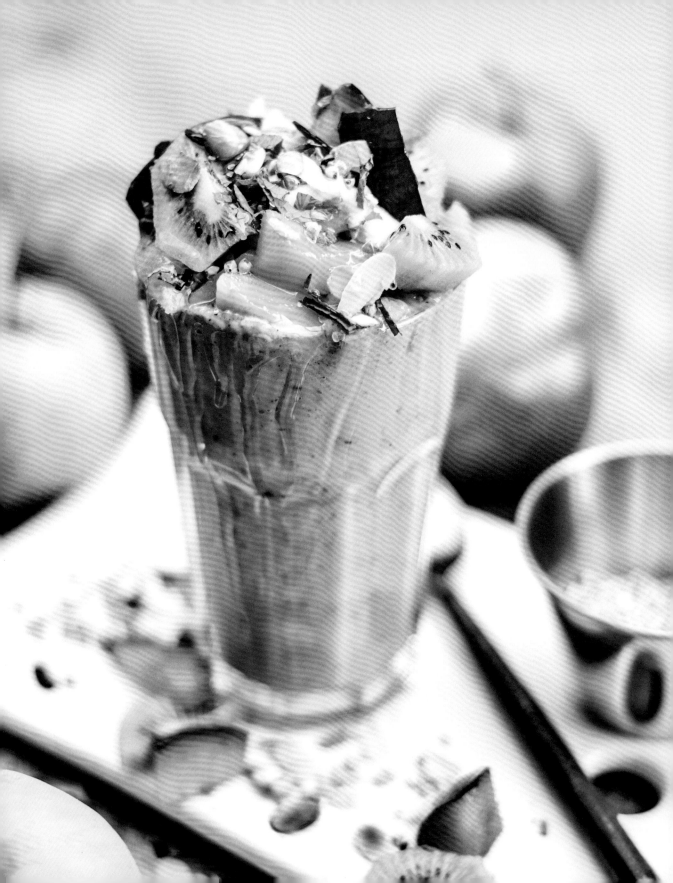

Mango Maca Protein Smoothie

Having smoothies for breakfast three to four times a week has done more than give us back time; they have boosted our energy levels, made us feel fuller for longer and helped us to drop kilos without losing important muscle. Smoothies also improve digestion, reduce bloating and keep things regular. If you haven't heard of the wonder plant maca, you are missing out. It has been used for centuries as a healing food, to boost energy and improve immunity. Maca is also said to have an adaptive response, which means that it helps our bodies adapt to stress. Its pleasant malt taste goes perfectly with mango in a smoothie. This drink is a wonderful superfood snack when you're having one of those hectic days.

SERVES 1

What's in it?

1 small handful of ice (if using fresh mango)

½ frozen, sliced banana

½ fresh mango or 1 cup (150g) frozen mango

1 scoop natural protein powder

1 cup (250ml) coconut water or coconut milk

1 tsp maca powder

1 tsp raw honey (optional)

1 tsp ground cinnamon

Put the ice, if using, banana, mango, protein powder, coconut water, maca powder, honey and cinnamon into a blender or food processor. Blitz until smooth and creamy, then serve.

Tips

Add more coconut water or milk, if you prefer a thinner consistency.

You can substitute the coconut water for almond milk, if you prefer.

Top with your favourite fruit and drizzle with honey.

Almond Mocha Smoothie

This is a smooth alternative to fruit smoothies, and there's a very good chance you'll want this nutty, chocolaty little beauty to replace your morning coffee – and maybe the afternoon one too. Chocolate and coffee are a match made in heaven, and, combined with almond milk and a little sweetness from the banana and dates, this mixture is a decadent smoothie to say the least. Don't be put off by the avocado. It brings a creamy texture to the smoothie and adds more good fats. This is definitely a treat smoothie.

SERVES 1

What's in it?

1 cup (250ml) almond milk

1 shot of espresso coffee

½ avocado, pitted, peeled and roughly chopped

½ banana, sliced

1 tbsp cacao

2–3 dried pitted dates or natural sweetener such as organic honey or maple syrup

1 small handful of ice

Put all the ingredients in a blender or food processor and blitz until smooth. Serve.

Tips

For a boost, add a scoop of natural protein powder.

Add more almond milk, if you prefer a thinner consistency.

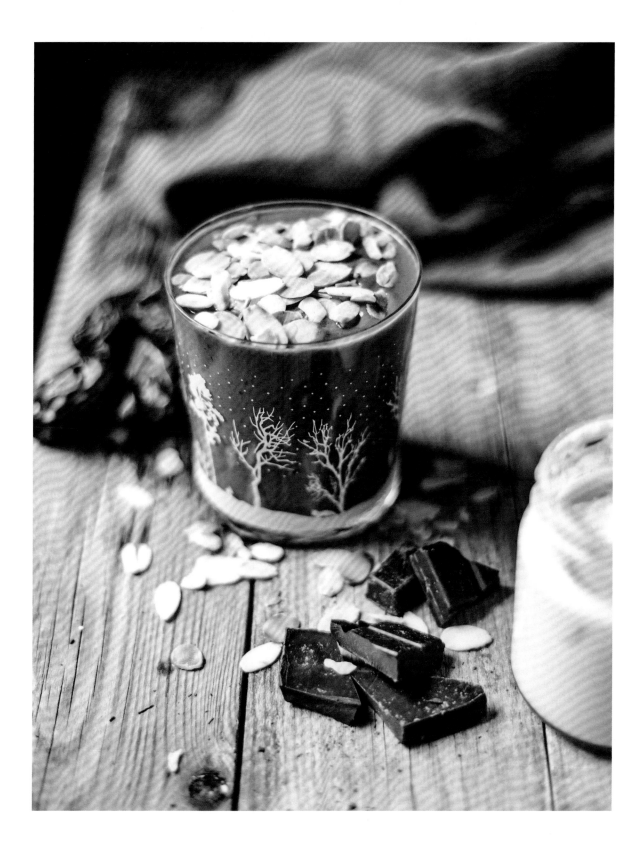

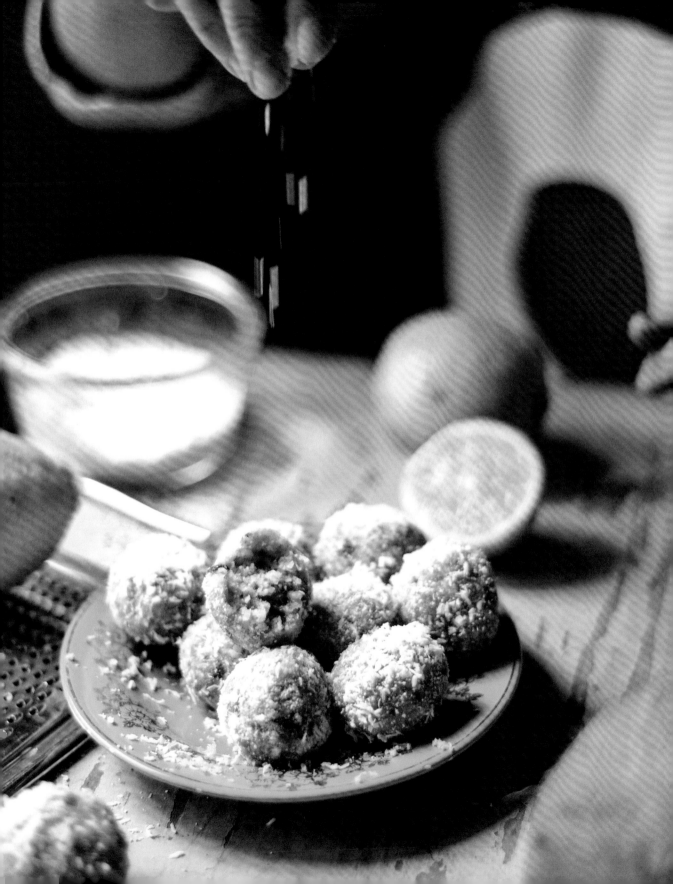

Cashew, Coconut and Lemon Protein Balls

Here is a tastebud delight that fits into your palm: protein balls that are perfect for little ones – and, of course, deserving mums too. We always have a batch of protein balls in the freezer, and we use a quality protein powder and nuts as a base for a quick protein hit. They taste just like an old-fashioned lemon slice without the nasty sugar.

MAKES 14

What's in it?

1 cup (120g) cashew nuts

¼ cup (35g) natural protein powder (optional)

5 dried pitted dates

¼ cup (50g) coconut oil, melted

1 tsp lemon juice

1 tsp lemon zest

1 tbsp desiccated coconut

Put the cashew nuts, protein powder and dates into a food processor and blitz until you get a fine consistency. Add the oil, lemon juice and zest, and blitz again until the ingredients start to clump together. If the ingredients are too dry and don't stick together, add a little water or more coconut oil.

Tip into a large bowl, then take small amounts at a time and roll into bite-sized balls. Put the desiccated coconut in a saucer and roll the balls in the coconut to coat completely. Store in an airtight container in the freezer for up to 2 weeks.

Tips

Slightly dampen your hands when rolling into balls to prevent the ingredients sticking.

If you don't have time to roll, press the ingredients into a baking tray lined with baking paper. Freeze to set, then remove and cut into small bars. Then re-freeze.

Simply Raw Choc Almond Slice

This treat fits perfectly with the healthy lifestyle you're aiming to achieve. And, as a bonus, it's a healthy and super-yummy alternative to cake in kids' lunch boxes too. Perfect for an occasional treat, this raw slice can be made in just 10 minutes. You can buy toasted almond meal (ground almonds) or pop it in the frying pan and toast it yourself. Even though this is not essential, it brings out the almond flavour. With the added dark chocolate on top, the kids think they are eating a chocolate bar. What a sneaky way to indulge in a healthy treat.

MAKES ABOUT 20 SQUARES

What's in it?

1 cup (100g) almond meal (ground almonds), toasted briefly in a frying pan

1 cup (130g) almonds, soaked in water overnight

5 dried pitted medjool dates

¼ cup (55g) tahini

¼ cup (50g) coconut oil, melted

1 tbsp rice malt syrup

1 tsp vanilla paste

Topping

85g dark, 70 per cent cocoa solids chocolate, melted

Line a 20 x 20 x 2.5cm square (or similar sized) tin or plastic container with baking paper.

Put the almond meal, soaked almonds and dates into a food processor and blitz until the almonds become fine and are mixed with the almond meal. Add the tahini, coconut oil, rice malt syrup and vanilla paste. Blitz again until the ingredients combine and clump together.

Remove and press evenly into the prepared tin, then freeze for approximately 2 hours or until set.

Meanwhile, melt the chocolate in a heatproof bowl over a pan of gently simmering water, making sure the base of the bowl doesn't touch the water. When fully melted, spread the chocolate evenly onto the almond base, then return to the freezer to set. Once set, remove from the tray and cut into small squares. Store in an airtight container in the freezer for up to two weeks (if you can resist them for that long!).

Tips

Line the tray with glad wrap/clingfilm: the base will lift out super-easy when removed from the tray.

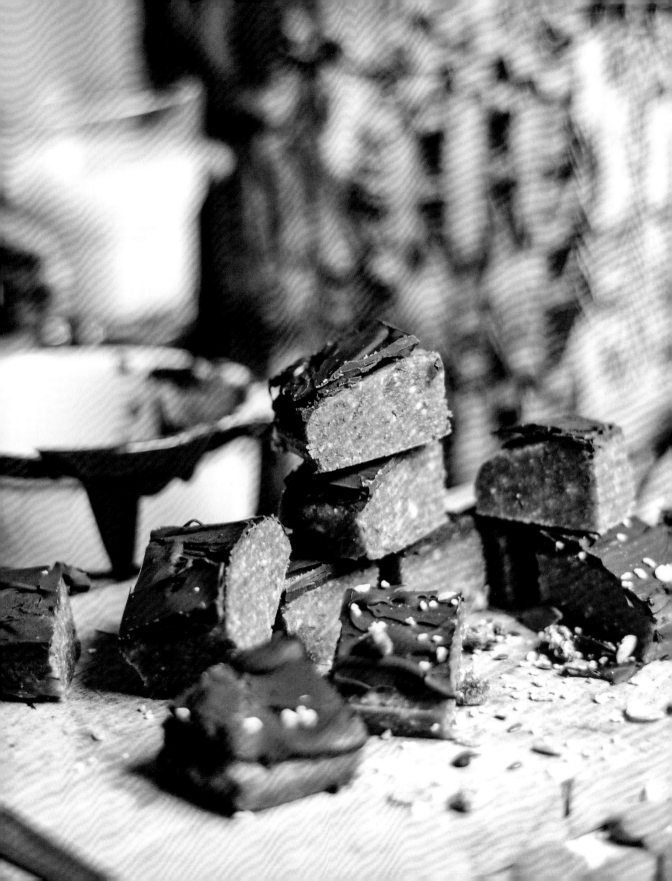

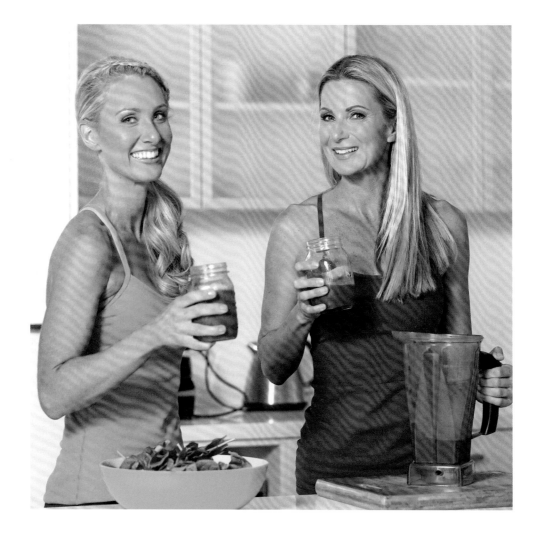

Added extras we wouldn't be without

Bone Broth

We are always on the lookout for inexpensive natural ways to improve our body inside and out. Looking and feeling younger has a lot to do with how we treat our body, especially what we put inside it. Drinking a cup of delicious old-fashioned bone broth works from the inside out to give you radiant skin and inner health. As we age, our collagen levels drop. Collagen gives our skin its elasticity, so we need to replace it. The collagen in bone broth comes from the bones and cartilage from beef, lamb or chicken – think of gran's homemade chicken soup. When the bones are cooked down, the collagen is released and turns into easily digestible gelatine. Bone broth has other amazing benefits: it helps to prevent wrinkles and sagging skin; it aids the digestion; it builds immunity; it is anti-inflammatory and it repairs muscle and joints.

What's in it?

1kg beef bones, a mixture of knuckle and marrow bone, large bones chopped – ask your butcher to do this

1 large onion, sliced

1 garlic clove, crushed

1 carrot, sliced

1 zucchini (courgette), sliced

4–8 cups (1–2 litres) filtered water (enough to cover the bones)

1 tbsp apple cider vinegar

sea salt and ground black pepper

Put the bones and vegetables in large pan or a slow cooker (hot pot), then pour in the water so that the bones are completely covered. Add the apple cider vinegar, and season with salt and pepper. Put the lid on and bring to the boil over a high heat if cooking in a pan, then reduce to a gentle simmer. If cooking in a slow cooker, set the slow cooker to Low. Cook the broth in the pan for 7 hours or in the slow cooker for 24–48 hours.

Remove the bones and drain the liquid through a sieve, discarding the vegetables. We like to store the broth in sealable glass jars in the fridge. Once cooled, you can remove the top layer of fat and use it for cooking.

Tips

You can also freeze the broth for up to 1 year. It's great to have on hand and use as stock in soups and casseroles, or simply store it in the fridge for up to 5 days and heat it up on the stove.

Kombucha

The ancient Chinese elixir probiotic drink, kombucha, is made from black or green tea, sugar and a SCOBY (symbiotic culture of bacteria or yeast). It is fermented for about ten days and, during the fermenting process, the SCOBY feeds off the sugar in the tea, decreasing the sugar content and turning the tea into a slightly sweet-tasting cider, which produces highly beneficial flora and probiotics. Your kids will love it. You can purchase the SCOBY online.

What's in it?

8 cups (2 litres) filtered water

2 black or green tea bags

1 cup (200g) raw organic sugar

1 SCOBY

1 cup (250ml) starter kombucha tea from a previous batch, or you can buy a small bottle from a health-food shop

You will also need

solid glass jar large enough to hold 8 cups (2 litres) boiling water

muslin cloth

rubber band

glass bottles with plastic lids to store the kombucha

wooden or plastic spoon (do not use metal to stir)

Boil the water in the kettle, pour into a large glass jar or jug and add the tea bags, then stir in the sugar. Allow the tea to cool to room temperature. Once cooled, remove the tea bags and put the SCOBY and starter kombucha into the jar or jug with the cooled tea and sugar. Cover the opening with muslin and secure with an elastic band.

Put the kombucha in a dark cupboard to ferment for about 10 days. We recommend that you taste test at day 8: the kombucha should be slightly sweet/bitter if it is ready. If your kombucha is still very sweet, return it to the cupboard for the full 10 days to ferment.

Remove your SCOBY and pour the kombucha into bottles, tighten the lids so that no air can escape. Put in the fridge to drink straight away or store in the cupboard. Store your SCOBY in a glass jar with enough kombucha liquid to totally submerge it. Cover and leave in a dark place until you are ready to make a new batch, or keep the cycle going by making a new batch every 10 days.

Start by drinking 1–2 small glasses (about 1¼ cups/300ml) a day, preferably before a meal.

Tips

Be careful not to leave the fermenting kombucha for too long, as it might taste very bitter, like vinegar. The warmer weather tends to ferment kombucha more quickly.

The benefits of kombucha

Kombucha is adaptive: it will work with your body to improve your digestion and help rebalance your gut flora, resulting in less bloating, a flatter stomach and an increased metabolism. Bad digestion will hamper fat loss and leave you feeling tired and sluggish, which can result in sugar cravings.

Kombucha's amazing health benefits include: improved digestion; reduced bloating; increased metabolism; a curb on sugar cravings; increased energy; improved immunity; clearer skin; it is anti-inflammatory; and it fights colds and stomach upsets (it's great for kids). Don't worry if you get stomach rumblings at the beginning. This is due to the bacteria in your stomach readjusting and improving the gut flora.

PART 3
The **Strong** Stuff

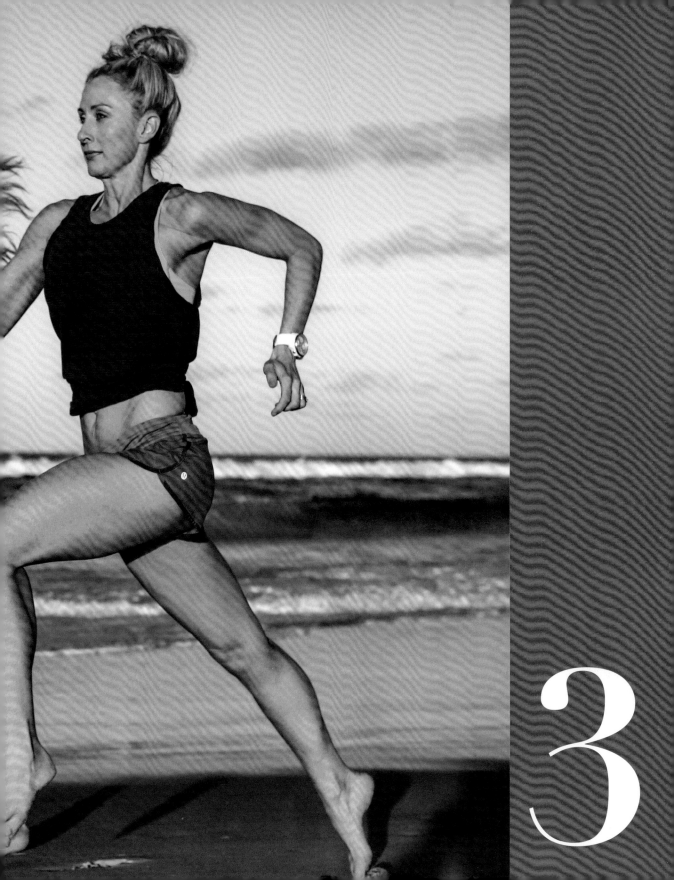

3

CHAPTER 6

Busy Mums Train Smart

Okay, here's the section you've probably been dreading. But don't worry, because getting into the physical stuff really doesn't have to be scary – and remember, we plan to make it as easy as possible for you.

There really isn't much point in trying to get into top shape if you're only going to look at either just eating healthy or just doing exercise alone. Exercise and food go hand in hand for becoming healthy, fit and happy. The last thing we want you to do is jump into an exercise or diet regime that you won't be able to maintain or that you feel is unrealistic. That's why we've crafted the Stay Strong Mummy Plan to suit your busy daily lifestyle, and we know that you'll be able to put it all together – even with the kids in tow.

The physical training and exercise we have in mind for you is realistic, achievable and it will suit your lifestyle, but first it's probably important that we go over some of the basics of why you need to focus on exercise as well as diet, and what kind of goals you should be setting when it comes to exercise.

Exercise is the vital physical stimulus for change and, as such, it should directly address our training goals. Typically, mummy training goals (exercise goals) should include:

• Fat loss – targeting the trouble areas of hips, tummy, legs, back and arms.

• Improved energy levels – to have more energy than is required to survive the daily grind; to have the energy to thrive.

• Improved strength – to have more strength than is required to survive the daily grind; to have the strength to thrive.

• Increased mobility – mobility allows our bodies to move in the way it was designed; to improve efficiency in the way we move and reduce the risk of injuries.

After much trial and error, injuries, unsustainable training programmes and fads, we've found the perfect training style for mums. The way we look and feel is very simply a consequence of our daily actions. We've made sure our training is an effective and efficient part of our day. It's important to note that prior to becoming mums, we were both far from world-class athletes. We've never been blessed with a lot of spare time, and we both had more than our fair share of emotional ups and downs. For this reason, our training is easily adapted to all levels of physical capabilities and it gives great results.

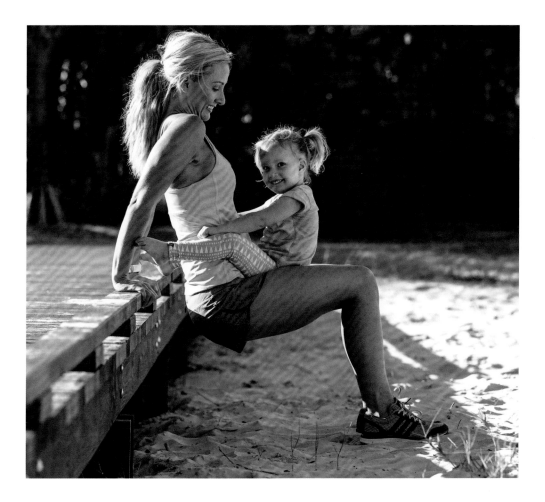

Since becoming mothers, we've both felt the need to be physically stronger and mentally more focused than we did when we were our pre-children selves. As mothers, we feel gifted with a natural strength, resilience and selflessness, which are constantly displayed by all mothers in the everyday activities of caring for our loved ones.

As mums, we often overlook ourselves in all aspects of life. It's ironic how mums can easily appreciate traits like strength and organisational skills in other mothers without acknowledging their own positive characteristics. Getting great results from training assists in releasing us from some of the emotional guilt associated with the few minutes of 'mummy time' required to achieve our goals.

To get started we will first look at a type of training that is extremely efficient and is made up of short, intense bursts of activity. It is called HIIT.

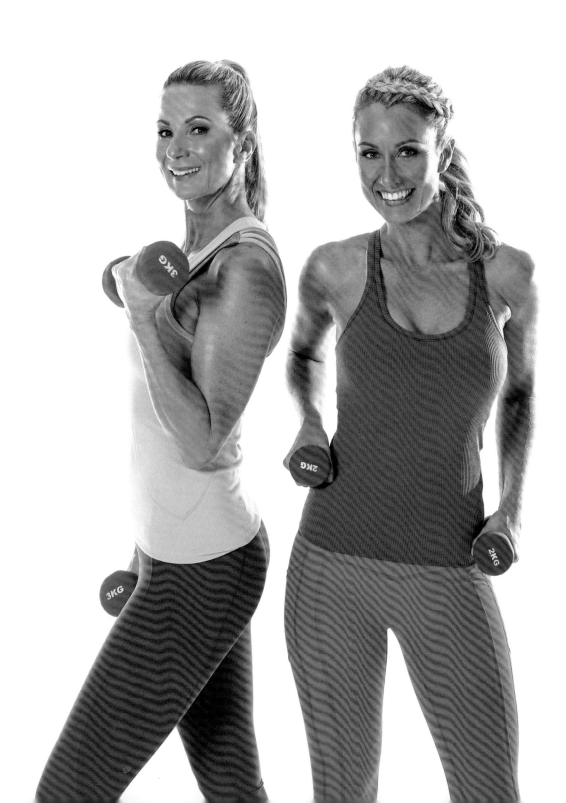

What is HIIT?

High-intensity interval training, otherwise referred to as HIIT, is circuit-style training that typically arranges four to eight goal-related exercises into a time-efficient workout. The exercise movements are the high-intensity workout periods – for example, 20 seconds – and are followed by short rest/recovery periods – for example 10 seconds.

HIIT exercises are placed in an order that will allow you to maintain maximum effort throughout the workout. Total training times are short (15–25 minutes), enabling a highly concentrated training effort and quality recovery from the sessions. The shorter and higher intensity workouts are invigorating and physically easier to recover from, making training far more sustainable and easy to adopt as a regular part of our lifestyles. Now you can see why HIIT is the perfect exercise programme for busy mums.

HIIT is equally effective practised in the gym as it is when carried out in your own backyard or living room, and you can quickly set up a HIIT session in just about any environment, thanks largely to the adaptability of the exercises. A session can be constructed for the pool, for a bike, when walking hills or at the beach. We jump at the opportunity to train with other Stay Strong Mummies in our area, too, and we team up for a partner or small group session. We love it and we're sure you'll love it too.

Why HIIT? The benefits specific to mums

You can burn unwanted body fat through high-intensity interval training – becoming a fat-burning furnace! The greater physical demand of the training maximises fat utilisation, which is largely attributable to the EPOC effect (excess post-exercise oxygen consumption). The EPOC effect is the approximate two-hour period after training during which the body expends energy and burns fat to return to its pre-exercise metabolic state. Clinical studies and trials have proven that there is between a 9 per cent and 20 per cent increase in fat loss compared to a traditional steady-state training session of 30–40 minutes on a treadmill, bike or through jogging. Just as importantly, with major health benefits for mums, HIIT reduces the risk of hypertension, heart disease, diabetes, arthritis and osteoporosis.

Specific training for mums The movements of the exercises, the total time of the workouts and the physical adaptations of the training are very specific to the needs of mums. The exercises replicate the demands of the everyday physical challenges in our lives: bend, twist, hold, push or pull – sometimes one or sometimes all at once. The combination of the physical demands on muscle use and the coordination of movements place a large metabolic demand on the body. This means we burn up many more calories in far less time.

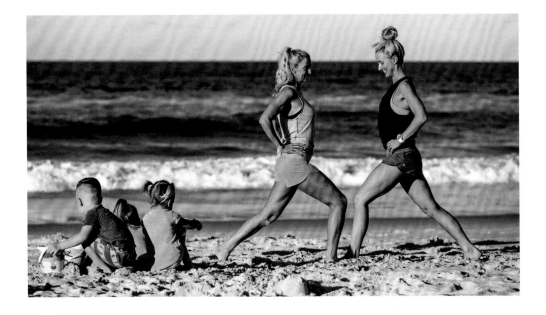

Sustainable training for mums We can already be under great stress. Our body does not distinguish between the stressors that cause stress hormones to be produced, whether they are as a result of daily thought-related worrying or the physical demands of exercise. Training sessions in excess of 45 minutes can contribute to stress, because they do not enable the body to effectively recover, and they will therefore negate much of the hard work of your training. HIIT, on the other hand, is sustainable, because while it stimulates adaptation towards our training goals, the adjustable variations allow for quality recovery; in other words, the ability to adjust total work time, work intensity, variation of movements and variation of work-to-recovery ratios according to individual needs. It's important to note here that we do have 45-minute sessions in our programme. These sessions are 45 minutes of *incidental activity*; that is, a lifestyle activity that you can build into your day, such as playing soccer in the park with the kids. These longer active sessions are supplementary but they are still an important part of the overall programme. It is training that can be disguised as a fun family event and assists with active recovery from your HIIT sessions, as well as progressing your overall fitness.

Training for all mums HIIT is beneficial for mums of *all* capabilities. The ability to adjust the physical demands of all exercises up or down makes this an effective training method, whether you're a beginner or an elite athlete. We regularly train with our husbands using the same workout design we've used for new clients on our Stay Strong Mummy groups.

The secret of HIIT

While there is undeniable science demonstrating the benefits of HIIT, its success is based on one very simple secret: having mental and physical commitment to the training.

Mental commitment: this means being present in the moment of exercise, embracing the positive effect you are in pursuit of and making every repetition count. Like anything in life, it is easy to be consumed by negative thoughts when we are fatigued – shake them off and embrace the challenge!

Physical commitment: once you have selected movements that are safely within your capabilities of timing, coordination and dynamic postural stability then go ahead and unleash the inner beast! You'll soon find you can shift that line in the sand of what was once your physical capability. Practicing HIIT will result in everyday life challenges, both mental and physical, becoming more tolerable.

Stay Strong Mummy – the recipe for HIIT success

There are three basic training methods that are usually followed to improve the body:

1 Strength-burst workouts Traditional strength training is the high mental (neural) and physical demand of training with heavy weights. This style of training improves our neural efficiency and enables us to shift heavy objects. Strength training is perfect for crafting lean, long muscles leading to a toned, sleek body.

2 Firm-body workouts Body-weight training is exercising using our own body weight as the resistance. The stress of body-weight training can improve our range of motion and mobility, as well as strength and body composition. Body-weight training is an extremely versatile and convenient way for busy mums to work out that won't put demands on the weekly budget.

3 Fat-blast workouts Cardiovascular training is body movement designed to keep the heart rate and oxygen consumption elevated for the duration of the session. In order to maintain constant movement, the stress of the activity is well within our capability, which allows for the longer training sessions.

One method with all the qualities of the above three:

Stay Strong Mummy HIIT is a fusion of all three training methods, which enables us to capitalise on all the positive benefits for mums.

Mummy Mantra

I work out for patience. I work out for clarity of mind

CHAPTER 7

Your Four-Week Fitness Plan

The Stay Strong Mummy Four-Week Fitness Plan gives you the structure you need to kick-start any thoughts you've had about getting active – or, if you're already training, it can provide a new direction for you to take. It's easy to set up, and the time efficiency of the programme will make home workouts a sustainable part of your busy mummy lifestyle.

Why we aim to be energy inefficient

The total time of the workouts ranges from 14 to 24 minutes. Each of the workouts is different, either by exercise or work-to-rest ratios. When training for fat loss, the number-one enemy of getting great results is *adaptation*. When we adapt to movements, workout times or workout intensities, we become very efficient (coordinated) in the way we move, and we end up requiring much less energy to move. Fat loss requires a lot of energy expenditure. Therefore, we need to train in a manner that is very *energy inefficient*. A constant variation of exercises, the continual adjustment of timing of work-to-rest periods and overall training time keeps us inefficient with our energy expenditure.

We've all trained in a way that has physically challenged us. Over time, we repeat the training and we end up less and less fatigued from what was once an incredible challenge. This classic example of adaptation is what we must avoid to continually get the best from our training effort and time.

Each training session is an opportunity to challenge us, remove obstacles and increase our own perception of our capabilities. We only ever compete against ourselves, and we are always committed and honest with our effort in the session.

Mummy Mantra

I am strong enough. I can do this. I deserve this

For effective recovery and better training performance, resist the urge to slump between sets, as it limits our breathing and reduces the ability of the working muscles to get rid of the 'waste products' built up from activity. Maintain a good posture and keep moving around. The duration of each exercise and rest between exercises will change over the weeks to maintain progressive overload, gradually building strength, improving stamina and stripping unwanted body fat.

Warm up

It's important that before any type of workout, we take the time to warm up and get ourselves physically and mentally prepared. There is a no more efficient way to warm up than to use the muscles and mimic the movements of what we are about to do. Simply perform six to eight slow repetitions of each exercise in the planned workout.

Put simply, the challenge will be the consistency to complete 16 sessions in four weeks, as this is the stimulus needed for a positive change. Before you start to doubt yourself, though, think about all the amazing achievements you've made so far in your journey as a mum. You really are amazing and you deserve to feel amazing all the time. This four-week exercise programme is exactly what you've been looking for in finding that newer, more vibrant you. Why wait? Today's a great time to start.

Active recovery

Active recovery means continually moving between sets. It keeps our blood pressure and heart rate elevated, which helps the blood to remove the build up of lactic acid in our working muscles. It will help you recover and perform better in the next set.

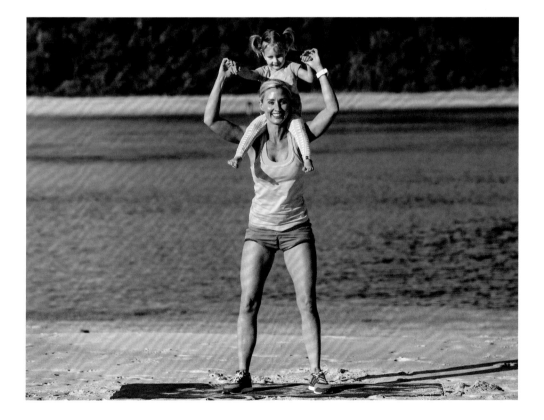

WEEK 1, SESSION 1

Fat-Blast Workout

Exercise	Time
1 Alternate Jump Lunge (page 176)	20 seconds
2 Rest	10 seconds
3 Push-Up (page 177)	20 seconds
4 Rest	10 seconds
5 Jump Squat (page 178)	20 seconds
6 Rest	10 seconds
7 Triceps Push-Up (page 179)	20 seconds
8 Rest	10 seconds
9 Mountain Climber (page 180)	20 seconds
10 Rest	10 seconds
11 Active recovery	1 minute

Total round time: 3 minutes 30 seconds

4 rounds – total workout: 14 minutes

WEEK 1, SESSION 2

Firm-Body Workout

Exercise	Time
1 Bulgarian Split Squat Left Leg (page 185)	20 seconds
2 Rest	10 seconds
3 Bulgarian Split Squat Right Leg (page 185)	20 seconds
4 Rest	10 seconds
5 Push-Up Turn Out (Alternating) (page 186)	20 seconds
6 Rest	10 seconds
7 Box Bridge (page 187)	20 seconds
8 Rest	10 seconds
9 Four-Point Alternate Superman (page 188)	20 seconds
10 Rest	10 seconds
11 Active recovery	1 minute

Total round time: 3 minutes 30 seconds

4 rounds – total workout: 14 minutes

WEEK 1, SESSION 3

Strength-Burst Workout

Exercise	Time
Exercise	*Time*
1 Dumbbell Squat to Shoulder Press (page 194)	20 seconds
2 Rest	10 seconds
3 Dumbbell Bent-Over Row (page 195)	20 seconds
4 Rest	10 seconds
5 Dumbbell Squat (page 196)	20 seconds
6 Rest	10 seconds
7 Renegade Row (page 197)	20 seconds
8 Rest	10 seconds
9 Straight-Leg Dumbbell Deadlift (page 198)	20 seconds
10 Rest	10 seconds
11 Active recovery	1 minute

Total round time: 3 minutes 30 seconds

4 rounds – total workout: 14 minutes

WEEK 1, SESSION 4

45 minutes of activity (see page 202)

WEEK 2, SESSION 1

Fat-Blast Workout

Exercise	Time
1 Sumo Jump Squat (page 181)	30 seconds
2 Rest	15 seconds
3 A-Frame Shoulder Press (page 182)	30 seconds
4 Rest	15 seconds
5 Flo Jo (left) (page 183)	30 seconds
6 Rest	15 seconds
7 Flo Jo (right) (page 183)	30 seconds
8 Rest	15 seconds
9 Elevated Triceps Push-Up (page 184)	30 seconds
10 Rest	15 seconds
11 Active recovery	1 minute

Total round time: 4 minutes 45 seconds

4 rounds – total workout: 19 minutes

WEEK 2, SESSION 2

Firm-Body Workout

Exercise	Time
1 Dips (page 189)	30 seconds
2 Rest	15 seconds
3 Box Jumps (page 190)	30 seconds
4 Rest	15 seconds
5 Superman Push-Up (page 191)	30 seconds
6 Rest	15 seconds
7 Alternate Step-Up (page 192)	30 seconds
8 Rest	15 seconds
9 Straight-Arm Plank (feet elevated) (page 193)	30 seconds
10 Rest	15 seconds
11 Active recovery	1 minute

Total round time: 4 minutes 45 seconds

4 rounds – total workout: 19 minutes

WEEK 2, SESSION 3

Strength-Burst Workout

Exercise	Time
1 Static Dumbbell Lunge (left leg) (page 199)	30 seconds
2 Rest	15 seconds
3 Static Dumbbell Lunge (right leg) (page 199)	30 seconds
4 Rest	15 seconds
5 Plank with Dumbbell Row (page 200)	30 seconds
6 Rest	15 seconds
7 Iron Cross (page 201)	30 seconds
8 Rest	15 seconds
9 Dumbbell Squat to Shoulder Press (page 194)	30 seconds
10 Rest	15 seconds
11 Active recovery	1 minute

Total round time: 4 minutes 45 seconds

4 rounds – total workout: 19 minutes

WEEK 2, SESSION 4

45 minutes of activity (see page 202)

Fat-Blast Workout

Exercise	Time
1 Alternate Jump Lunge (page 176)	20 seconds
2 Rest	10 seconds
3 Push-Up (page 177)	20 seconds
4 Rest	10 seconds
5 Jump Squat (page 178)	20 seconds
6 Rest	10 seconds
7 Triceps Push-Up (page 179)	20 seconds
8 Rest	10 seconds
9 Mountain Climber (page 180)	20 seconds
10 Rest	10 seconds
11 Active recovery	1 minute

Total round time: 3 minutes 30 seconds

4 rounds – total workout: 14 minutes

WEEK 3, SESSION 2

Firm-Body Workout

Exercise	Time
1 Bulgarian Split Squat (left leg) (page 185)	20 seconds
2 Rest	10 seconds
3 Bulgarian Split Squat (right leg) (page 185)	20 seconds
4 Rest	10 seconds
5 Push-Up Turn Out (alternating) (page 186)	20 seconds
6 Rest	10 seconds
7 Box Bridge (page 187)	20 seconds
8 Rest	10 seconds
9 Four-Point Alternate Superman (page 188)	20 seconds
10 Rest	10 seconds
11 Active recovery	1 minute

Total round time: 3 minutes 30 seconds

4 rounds – total workout: 14 minutes

WEEK 3, SESSION 3

Strength-Burst Workout

Exercise	Time
1 Dumbbell Squat to Shoulder Press (page 194)	20 seconds
2 Rest	10 seconds
3 Dumbbell Bent-Over Row (page 195)	20 seconds
4 Rest	10 seconds
5 Dumbbell Squat (page 196)	20 seconds
6 Rest	10 seconds
7 Renegade Row (page 197)	20 seconds
8 Rest	10 seconds
9 Straight-Leg Dumbbell Deadlift (page 198)	20 seconds
10 Rest	10 seconds
11 Active recovery	1 minute

Total round time: 3 minutes 30 seconds

4 rounds – total workout: 14 minutes

WEEK 3, SESSION 4

45 minutes of activity (see page 202)

WEEK 4, SESSION 1

Fat-Blast Workout

Exercise	Time
1 Sumo Jump Squat (page 181)	40 seconds
2 Rest	20 seconds
3 A-Frame Shoulder Press (page 182)	40 seconds
4 Rest	20 seconds
5 Flo Jo (left) (page 183)	40 seconds
6 Rest	20 seconds
7 Flo Jo (right) (page 183)	40 seconds
8 Rest	20 seconds
9 Elevated Triceps Push-Up (page 184)	40 seconds
10 Rest	20 seconds
11 Active recovery	1 minute

Total round time: 6 minutes

4 rounds - total workout: 24 minutes

Firm-Body Workout

Exercise	Time
1 Dips (page 189)	40 seconds
2 Rest	20 seconds
3 Box Jumps (page 190)	40 seconds
4 Rest	20 seconds
5 Superman Push-Up (page 191)	40 seconds
6 Rest	20 seconds
7 Alternate Step-Up (page 192)	40 seconds
8 Rest	20 seconds
9 Straight-Arm Plank (feet elevated) (page 193)	40 seconds
10 Rest	20 seconds
11 Active recovery	1 minute

Total round time: 6 minutes

4 rounds - total workout: 24 minutes

WEEK 4, SESSION 3

Strength-Burst Workout

Exercise	Time
1 Static Dumbbell Lunge (left leg) (page 199)	40 seconds
2 Rest	20 seconds
3 Static Dumbbell Lunge (right leg) (page 199)	40 seconds
4 Rest	20 seconds
5 Plank with Dumbbell Row (page 200)	40 seconds
6 Rest	20 seconds
7 Iron Cross (page 201)	40 seconds
8 Rest	20 seconds
9 Dumbbell Squat to Shoulder Press (page 194)	40 seconds
10 Rest	20 seconds
11 Active recovery	1 minute

Total round time: 6 minutes

4 rounds - total workout: 24 minutes

WEEK 4, SESSION 4

45 minutes of activity (see page 202)

CHAPTER 8

The Stay Strong Mummy Exercises

In this section you'll find our step-by-step guide to performing the exercises. It's important to use the correct technique when performing our workouts, as this ensures that you are doing them effectively and efficiently, which will help you achieve the results that you're after. We recommend that you review each movement prior to doing the set, even if you're a seasoned pro.

Alternate Jump Lunge

Start in a running position, both legs with knees bent at 90 degrees. Jump, driving up through the front leg for good vertical height, and reverse the leg positions from front to back while in the air. Ensure that the landing is soft with control through the new front leg, lowering the new back knee down to a stable starting position, and repeat.

Tip

The front leg is the working leg with a demand for power to jump and then to control the landing speed. The rear leg is primarily used for balance during the exercise.

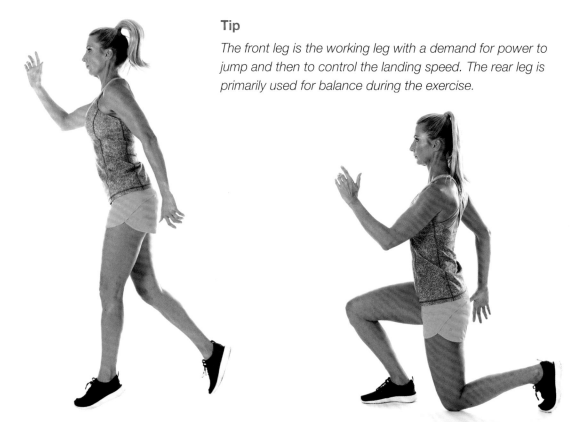

Push-Up

Begin in plank position with straight arms, hands set outside shoulder width. With a controlled bend at the elbows, lower the chest towards the ground and pivot from your toes. Only descend as deep as you can while maintaining control of the movement and your posture. (No shrugging shoulders or sagging lower back.) Push evenly through both hands to return to the starting position.

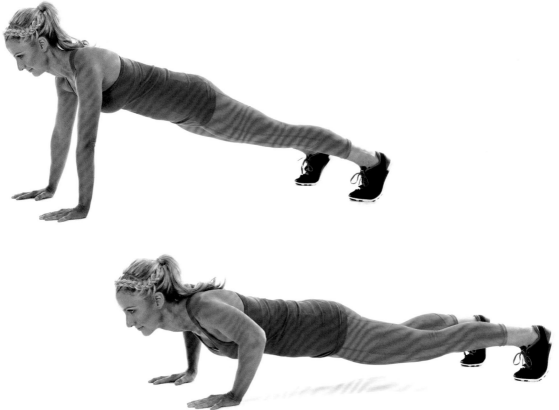

Tip

Invest in push-up handles if your wrists don't like the pressure placed on them during the exercise. To make the exercise easier, work with your hands on an elevated platform like a bench, chair or table.

Jump Squat

Your body weight should be even on both feet as you lower yourself into a position ready to jump. Only drop as deep as the mobility at your hips, knees and ankles will allow, arms reached forward for balance without slumping in the spine. Jump evenly off both legs, pulling your arms forcefully down to your side for added power. Land evenly on soft feet, knees slightly bent, and control the landing speed back to the starting position with arms reaching out the front for balance and control.

Tip

It's just as important to concentrate on landing control and balance as it is to focus on the power of the jump.

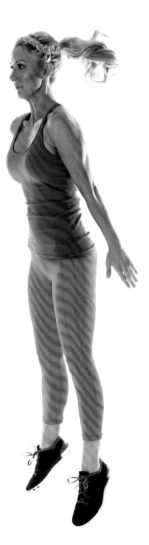
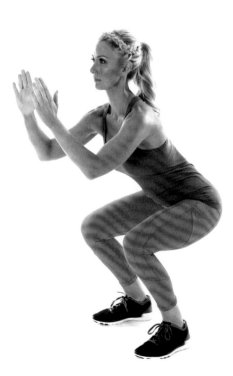

Triceps Push-Up

Begin in plank position with straight arms, hands placed at shoulder width, or closer, for emphasis on the triceps and shoulders. Have a controlled bend at the elbows (pointing backwards to your feet), lowering your chest towards the ground and pivoting from your toes. Only descend as deep as you can while maintaining control of the movement and your posture. (No shrugging shoulders or sagging lower back.) Push evenly through both hands to return to the starting position.

Tip

Keep your shoulder blades set down and back for postural strength and stability in the upper back.

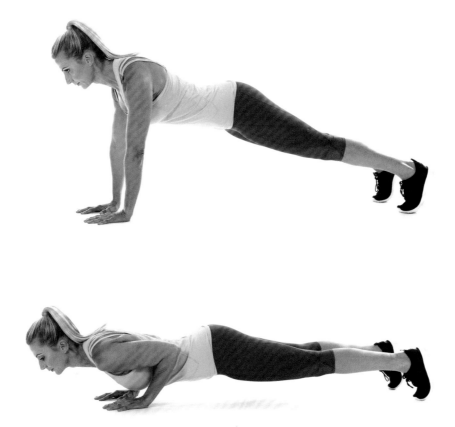

Mountain Climber

Start in a plank position, your hands a little wider than your shoulders. Activate the stabilising muscles in your trunk, focusing on always maintaining a neutral spine.

Alternately drive knees forward, each time landing on the ball of your front foot. Alternate your legs as quickly as possible while maintaining control through the trunk.

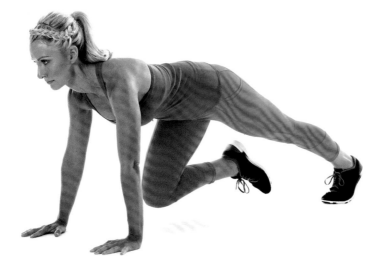

Tip

Your range will depend on your mobility and flexibility. Always keep a long neutral spine and level hips. Stay working safely within your range of movement.

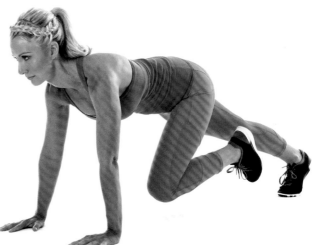

Sumo Jump Squat

Start with your feet wider than shoulder width. Your body weight should be even on both feet as you lower yourself into a position ready to jump. Only drop as deeply as your mobility at the hips, knees and ankles will allow – arms reached forward for balance, without slumping in the spine. Jump evenly off both legs, pulling your arms forcefully down to your sides for added power. Land with soft feet, knees slightly bent, and control the landing speed back to the starting position with arms reaching out front for control and balance.

Tip

Avoid landing on stiff, straight legs. For best results land softly, catching your bodyweight with your knees already bent, and control the deceleration back to starting position for the next jump.

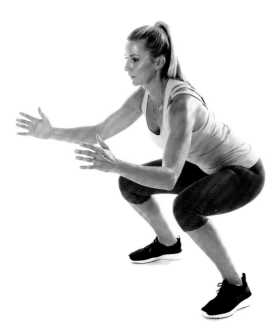
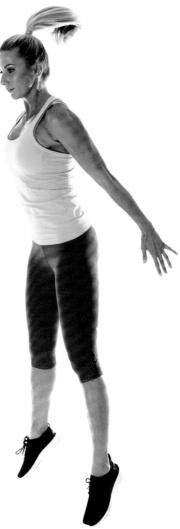

A-Frame Shoulder Press

Start in a downward-dog position creating an A-frame with hands shoulder-width apart and pressed firmly into the mat. Keeping your neck long, bend your elbows, lowering your head towards the mat as far as you have control of the movement and your posture. Straighten your elbows back to the starting position. Keep your shoulders down and away from your ears.

Tip

Look through your legs; keep your legs tight and the hips high. Slightly bend your knees if you have tight hamstrings.

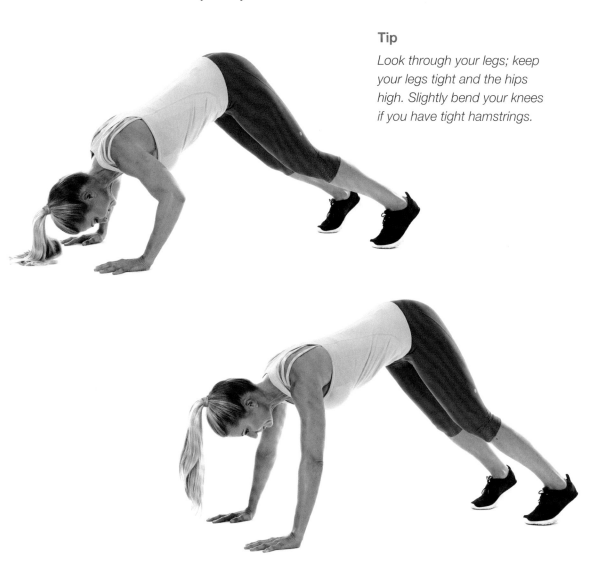

Flo Jos

Stand and maintain a strong running position with the front leg constantly grounded with a soft bent knee. The rear leg thrusts forwards and then backwards, mimicking a running action in continuous motion. Your arms should move as if you are running.

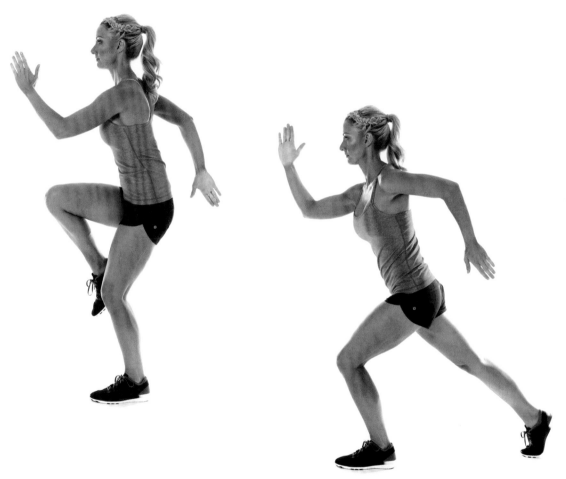

Tip

To increase the intensity of the exercise, increase the tempo and range of movement in the back leg.

Elevated Triceps Push-Up

Place your hands shoulder-width or closer on a stable elevated surface, such as a bench, low table, chair or step. Control the bend at the elbows (pointing backwards to your feet) lowering your chest towards the surface and pivoting from your toes. The elevated surface should allow you a much-increased range of movement so that you can maintain control of the movement and good posture. (No shrugging shoulders or sagging lower back.) Push evenly through both hands to return to the starting position.

Tip

Keep your shoulder blades set down and back for postural strength and stability in the upper back.

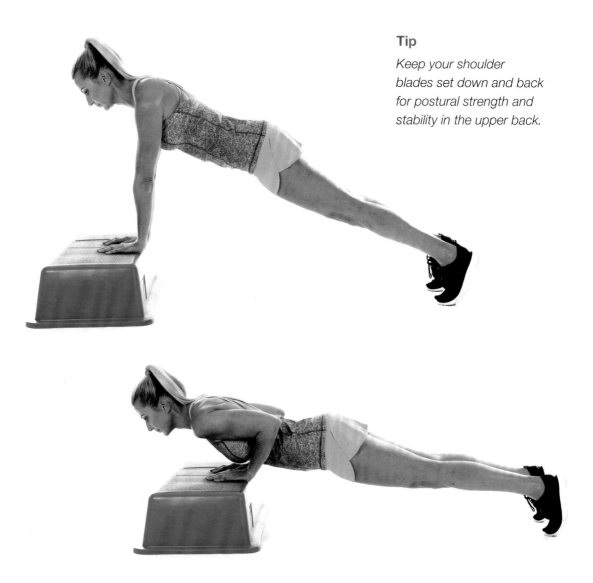

Bulgarian Split Squat

Stand in a lunge position. Focus on your balance and force through the front foot, as this is the working leg. The back foot should be placed on an elevated surface, such as a bench, step or ball. Interlock your fingers and place your hands behind your head without pulling your head forward. Bend your front leg until the back knee lightly touches the ground. Drive your weight through the heel of the front foot to return back to the starting position.

Tip

Keep your hips squarely facing forward at all times. The exercise movement is up and down, not forwards and backwards. Resist slumping forward from the hips, as this lessens the intensity of the exercise.

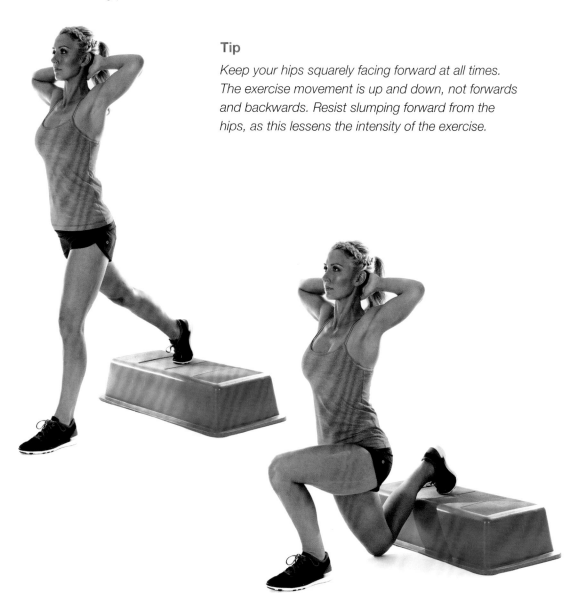

Push-Up Turn Out (alternating)

Begin in plank position with straight arms, hands set outside shoulder width. Make a controlled bend at the elbows, lowering your chest towards the ground and pivoting from your toes. Only descend as deeply as you can while maintaining control of the movement and your posture. (No shrugging shoulders or sagging lower back.) As you push away from the ground, rotate out to the side, one hand down making a T-shape with the other arm extended, feet stacked one on top of the other. Control the lateral plank position for 2 seconds before rolling back, repeating the push-up action and lateral plank on the opposite side.

Tip

When holding the lateral plank, ensure that your hips and shoulders are aligned with a neutral spine. You want to avoid your hips rolling out and your chest rolling in.

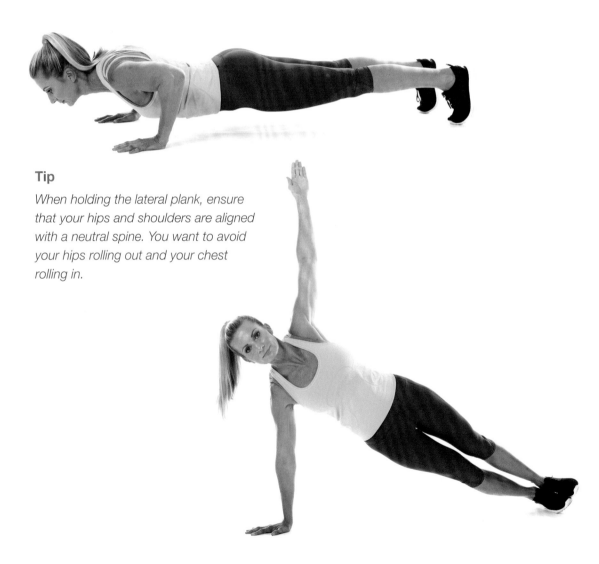

Box Bridge

Lying on your back, place your feet on an elevated platform, such as a step, bench or ball, with a 90-degree bend in your knees. With the driving force through your heels, lift your hips from the ground until your body is aligned in a straight line from your knees to your hips to your shoulders. Lower your hips back to the ground and repeat the movement.

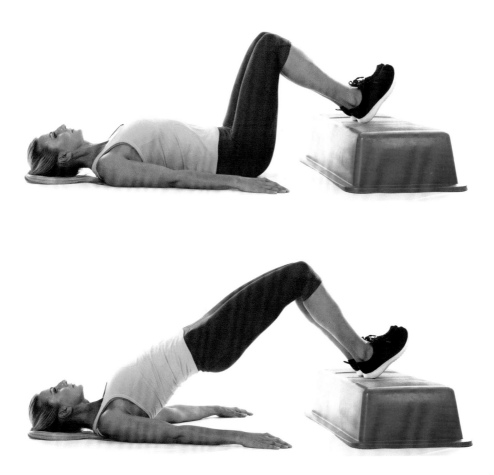

Tip

For maximum glute activation, imagine you are using your butt cheeks to squeeze and pull a tissue out the top of its box each time you lift your hips.

Four-Point Alternate Superman

Start with your weight evenly distributed on your hands and knees, and always be conscious of holding a neutral spine. At the same time, reach forward with your right arm and kick straight back with your left leg. Hold the position for 2 seconds, then return to the starting position. Now alternate sides: at the same time, reach forward with your left arm and kick straight back with your right leg. Hold the position for 2 seconds, then return to the starting position and alternate continuously.

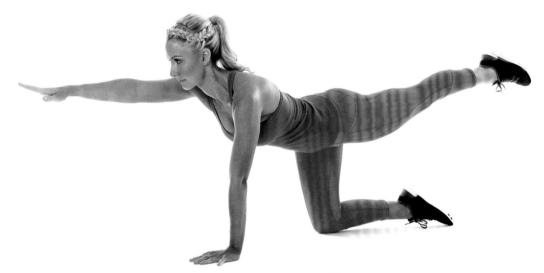

Tip

Avoid twisting in the trunk. If you were to lay a broomstick across your upper back and another across your lower back, they should not tip off.

Dips

Set your hands shoulder-width apart on an elevated surface, such as a chair or bench. Your legs should be bent at 90 degrees for the easiest load *or* legs straight and your bodyweight on your heels (or legs elevated) for maximum load on triceps and shoulders. While always maintaining a neutral spine, bend your elbows with control to a depth that you are safely able to straighten your arms and return back to the starting position.

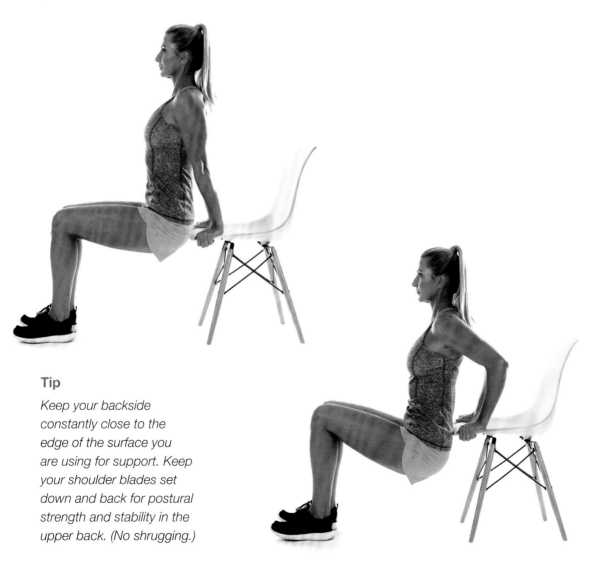

Tip

Keep your backside constantly close to the edge of the surface you are using for support. Keep your shoulder blades set down and back for postural strength and stability in the upper back. (No shrugging.)

Box Jumps

Select an elevated surface or platform with a height that will challenge your energy levels but is safely within your jumping-height capabilities. Jump evenly off both feet using your arms for assistance. Land simultaneously on both feet with soft bent knees. Jump backwards off the platform. Control your landing speed, descending smoothly back to the starting position with your arms out in front and your legs in position to repeat the effort.

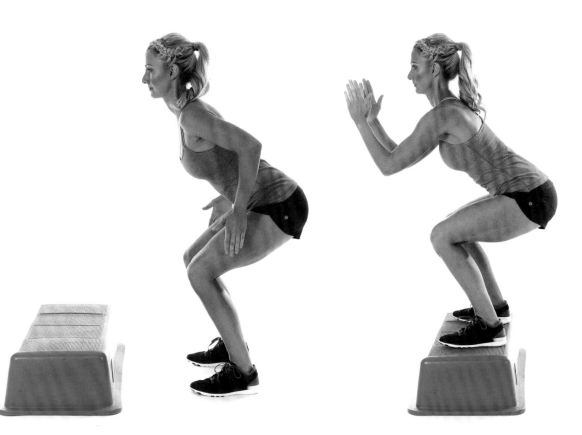

Tip

If you become excessively fatigued and it's affecting your control,
adjust to stepping off the platform back down to the starting position.

Superman Push-Up

Begin in plank position with straight arms, hands set outside shoulder width. With a controlled bend at the elbows, lower your chest all the way to the ground, pivoting from your toes. Reach your arms forwards, like superman, then return your hands to the starting position. Push-up, maintaining a neutral spine, with control of your posture from your hands to your toes.

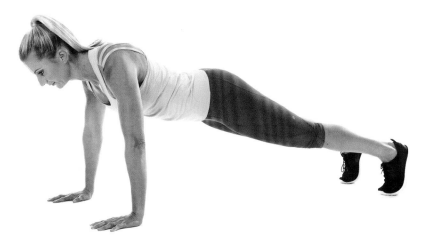

Tip

Don't allow your lower back to sag, and don't shrug your shoulders as you lower your chest to the ground.

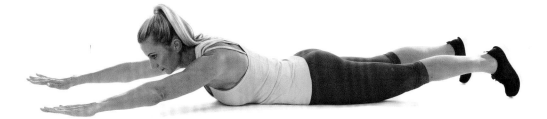

Alternate Step-Up

Place your left foot on an elevated platform, such as a bench or step. Focus strength and control through your left foot as you step up with the right foot to touch beside the left and then straight back to the ground. Concentrate on the left leg controlling the speed of the right foot as it descends back to the ground. Bring the left foot back to the ground. Now alternate. Place your right foot on the elevated platform. Focus your strength and control through the right foot as you step up with the left foot to touch beside the right and then straight back to the ground. Concentrate on the right leg controlling the speed of the left foot as it descends back to the ground. Bring the right foot back to the ground.

Continuously alternate, working your legs through the work period.

Tip

Use your arms in a running action to assist with the exercise. Try not to slump forward, as it will take working stress out of the working leg.

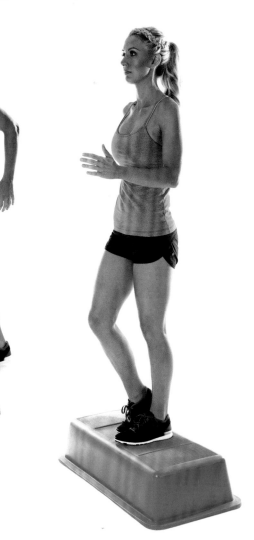

Straight-Arm Plank (feet elevated)

Adopt a plank position with your shoulders directly over your hands and your toes on an elevated platform, such as a bench, seat or step. Maintain a neutral spine and stay conscious of keeping your hips level at all times.

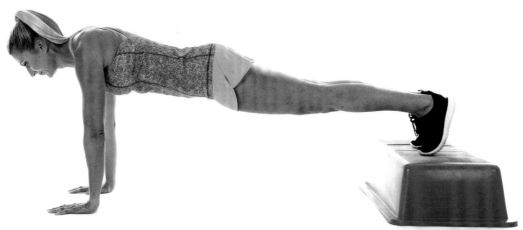

Tip

Increase the elevation to increase the demand of the exercise. Keep your shoulder blades down and retracted at all times.

Dumbbell Squat to Shoulder Press

Ensure your bodyweight is even on both feet, dumbbells in hand at shoulder height. Only drop as deeply as your mobility will allow at the hips, knees and ankles. Your elbows should be pointing forwards for balance, without slumping in the spine. Stand up evenly on both feet with emphasis through your heels. At the top of the squat, shoulder-press the dumbbells, then bring the dumbbells back to the shoulders, and repeat.

Tip

This exercise can burn! When you become experienced with controlling the movements and maintaining good posture, increase the tempo of the exercise for maximum energy expenditure. You can add a chair to assist with squat depth.

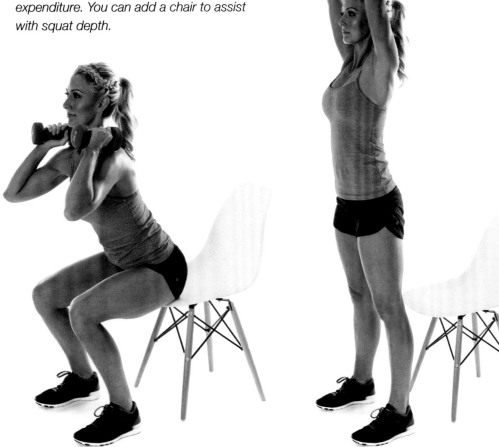

Dumbbell Bent-Over Row

Stand leaning forwards from your hips (at about 45 degrees) with your knees bent.

Ensure you maintain a neutral spine and keep your ribcage lifted and your shoulders down away from your ears. With the dumbbells in your hands, the arms should hang straight to the floor. The rowing action should be controlled in both directions.

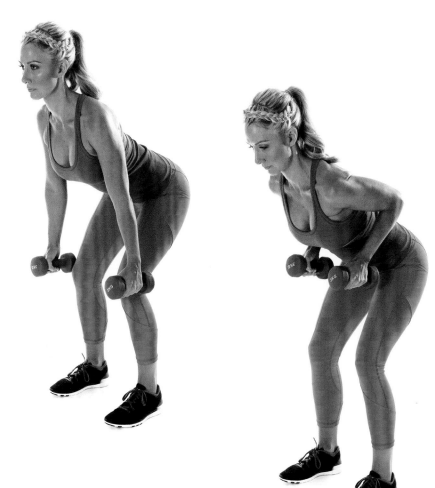

Tip

Your elbows should brush your sides. Shoulder stability and postural strength come from squeezing the shoulder blades back and together on every repetition.

Dumbbell Squat

Stand with dumbbells in your hands and your hands directly by your sides with your bodyweight evenly on both feet. As you descend, only drop as deeply as the mobility at your hips, knees and ankles will safely allow. Maintain a neutral spine, without slumping in the upper back or shrugging your shoulders. Stand up with your weight evenly distributed on both feet, driving extra force through your heels.

Tip

Keep the dumbbells constantly at your side for maximum load. Keep your eyes forward and your ribcage lifted as you stand in the squat.

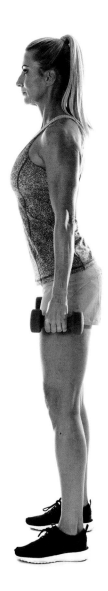
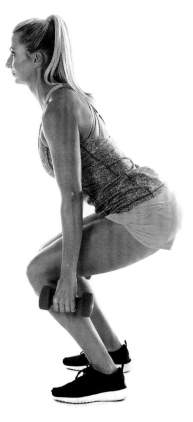

Renegade Row

Hold the dumbbells in your hands based on the ground and shoulder-width apart. Your hands should have thumbs forward, holding a plank at the top of the push-up position. Maintain the plank while alternately lifting the dumbbells with your elbow, brushing your side in a one-arm rowing action. After completing a row on each arm, perform one push-up and repeat the cycle.

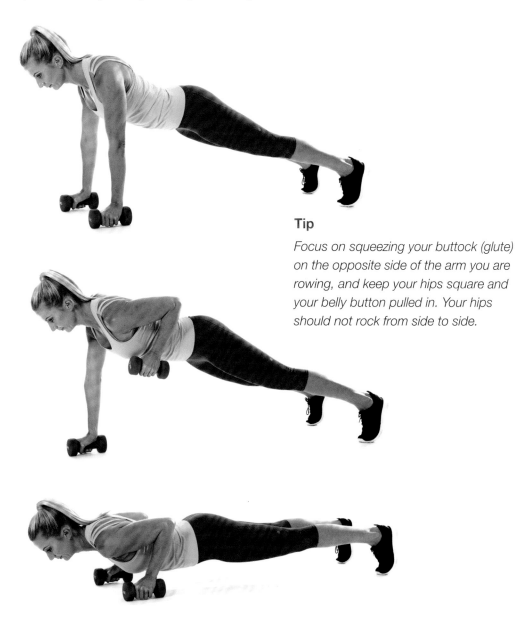

Tip

Focus on squeezing your buttock (glute) on the opposite side of the arm you are rowing, and keep your hips square and your belly button pulled in. Your hips should not rock from side to side.

Straight-Leg Dumbbell Deadlift

Stand with your feet hip-width apart and hold dumbbells with an overhand grip, resting them on the front of your thighs. Hinge forwards from the hips, lowering the dumbbells with straight arms, as close as you can get to your toes while keeping a perfectly neutral spine. Don't allow your back to round; keep your legs straight without locking out at the knees.

Concentrate on activating your glutes and hamstrings. Squeeze your glutes as you come back up to the starting position.

Tip

To keep this exercise safe and focused on the glutes/hamstrings, don't allow your back to round over. The exercise can feel like an active hamstring stretch.

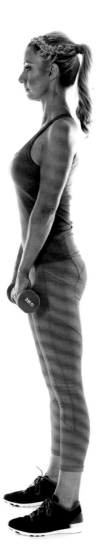
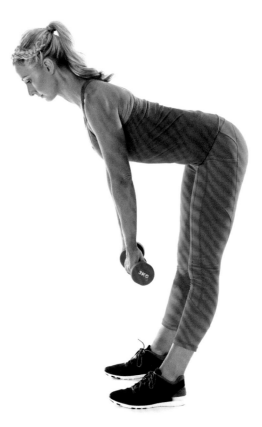

Static Dumbbell Lunge

Stand in a lunge position with the dumbbells in your hands and held in line with your hips at all times. Control and force is generated through the front foot of the working leg. Rest on the toes of your back foot, which is in place for balance and control. Bend the knee of your front leg until the back knee lightly touches the ground, then drive the weight through the heel of the front foot to return to the starting position.

Tip

Keep your hips facing squarely forward at all times. The exercise movement is up and down. Don't shift the dumbbells forwards and backwards; keep the load at the hips at all phases of the exercise. Resist slumping forward from the hips or rounding the upper back.

Plank with Dumbbell Row

Hold the dumbbells in your hands based on the ground and shoulder-width apart. Your hands should have the thumbs forward, holding a plank at the top of a push-up position. Maintain the plank while continuously lifting the dumbbells, with your elbows at your sides, in an alternating one-arm rowing action.

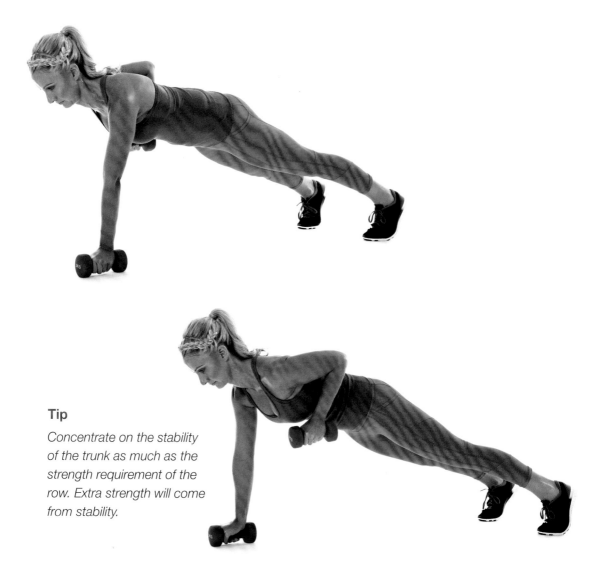

Tip

Concentrate on the stability of the trunk as much as the strength requirement of the row. Extra strength will come from stability.

Iron Cross

Start with your feet shoulder-width apart, dumbbells in hand and arms extended at shoulder level in a crucifix position. Your bodyweight should be even on both feet. As you descend, only drop as deeply as the mobility at your hips, knees and ankles will safely allow. Simultaneously bring your arms together out in front, maintaining a neutral spine. (No slumping in the upper back or shrugging your shoulders.) Stand up with your weight evenly distributed on both feet, driving extra force through your heels and opening your arms, returning to the crucifix position at the top of the movement.

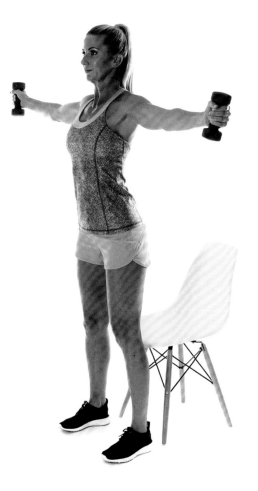

Tip

For a greater challenge, start with dumbbells together and open to crucifix position as you descend in the squat action. Only progress if you're capable of maintaining good posture throughout the movement. You can add a chair to help with squat depth.

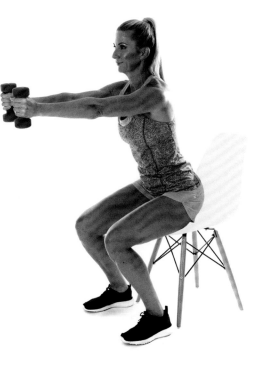

Suggested 45-minute cardio workouts

Cardio is an essential part of improving your fitness. As, it will help you to speed up your journey towards being fit and healthy. Most of our Plan exercises can be performed at home, but cardio might be easier for you to achieve in an open space, such as going for a walk or a run in the park. Obviously, this means having the kids in tow when you do your cardio, but they will usually find a trip to the big wide world as stimulating as you will. So get brave and get out – it's exactly what you need!

Here are some examples of how you can incorporate some cardio into your busy-mummy life:

• A 45-minute walk, bike ride or swim – they are all great for some family exercise.

• Sprints (at the park with the kids): 20 seconds sprinting and 10 seconds rest, for 8 rounds.

• Walk/run with the stroller. This is great if you're new to running and want to increase the length of your runs. Start off jogging for 45 seconds, then walk for 1 minute; repeat for 15 minutes. Then try running for 1 minute, walking for 1 minute; repeat for the next 15 minutes. For the final 15 minutes, try running for 2–3 minutes and walking for 1 minute – or slow down to a pace which you can maintain for the last 15 minutes while keeping your heart rate up. A good indication that you are maintaining intensity is that you cannot carry on a conversation while on the move.

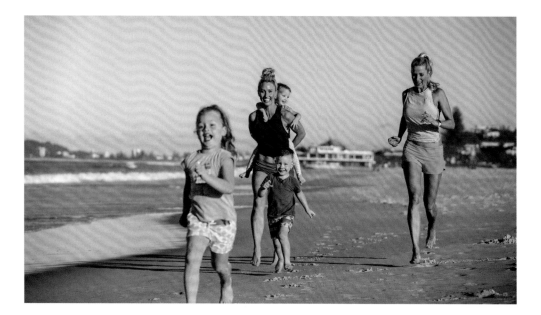

Remember: cardio is an optional extra to the Plan. If on some weeks you can fit it in, that's great; if on other weeks, you can't, don't stress about it. If you can do it every week, go for it. The added cardio session will help to speed up your weight loss. You can choose any of the workouts, but try to mix it up so that you're not doing the same thing every week.

How to make time to exercise

- Schedule your workouts into your day in the same way that you schedule an appointment to meet a friend for coffee.
- Set a routine – even if you start exercising for just one day per week, it's a start!
- Set the alarm 30 minutes earlier than usual.
- Have your workout gear, water bottle and so on, ready to go.
- Prep the night before: know exactly what exercise routine you are going to do the next day.
- Make your workout a priority, then plan your day around it.
- Lose the guilt on making time for yourself.
- Walk and talk on your next coffee date, instead of sitting and chatting.
- Use the time while you're waiting for your child at afterschool activities to go for a jog or walk. Find a park close by and do a 15-minute workout. Ask other mums to join you.
- If you're at the beach or in a park, play. Have a go on the monkey bars, play chase with the kids and practise cartwheels. Victoria is 45 and learned to do her first ever handstand two years ago.
- If you have young babies or infants, workout while they sleep. Your chores can wait for 15 minutes.
- If your babies are awake, set them up on a bouncer next to you and let them watch you jump around. If your jumping around upsets the babies, don't quit – just try again later.
- If your baby enjoys being in the stroller, go for a walk, but incorporate some HIIT into your walk by doing walking lunges and some jump squats while you rock the stroller. Or run with your stroller in intervals.

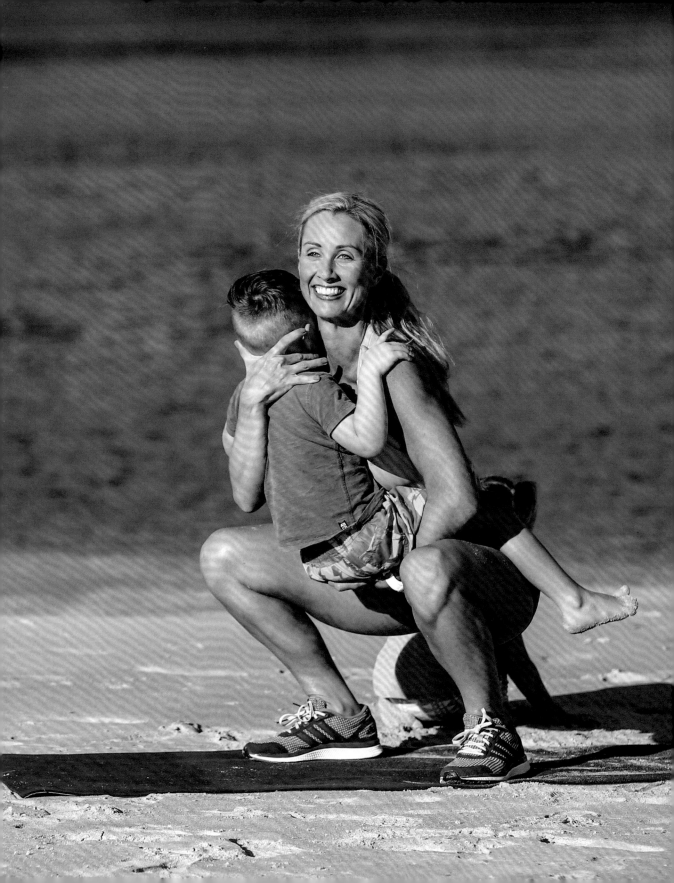

How to incorporate your children into your exercise routine

As a mother, there is generally no place like home, particularly when you have younger children. It's where most of your routine and daily happenings must take place in order to have a harmonious and balanced family life. There are other obvious benefits to working out at home too – such as wearing your favourite sloppy sweat pants and making the kids laugh out loud with the noises you make while you exercise. If it's convenient to be at home with your kids, then it's likely it will also be convenient for you to fit in a daily exercise routine at home too – once you know how.

Finding the time and energy to workout at home on a regular basis can prove challenging if you don't have someone else to motivate or encourage you, and that makes it even more important to find the right exercise routine that fits in with your busy lifestyle.

If having a babysitter around while you sweat it out is not an option, don't fret. You'll probably find that both you and the kids are likely to feel more relaxed at home than you would if you were to put the children in a crèche while you workout in a gym.

That's where we come in. Whether you've got a big backyard or a small area at the end of your bed, there is always room for a workout, and there are ways you can make a regular exercise routine not only achievable but also enjoyable. You really don't have to get to the gym to get your exercise in, nor do you have to purchase expensive exercise equipment.

The Stay Strong Mummy Plan gives you all the information, tips and know-how you'll need, so you can master your exercise routine and finesse your techniques. Before long, you'll be confident and wanting to involve the rest of the family. Whether they're watching you from a pram, sitting on a mat enjoying a snack, walking around you or riding their bike, it's a wonderful thing for your kids to see mummy living and breathing a healthy and active lifestyle.

'There are other obvious benefits to working out at home too – such as wearing your favourite sloppy sweat pants and making the kids laugh out loud with the noises you make while you exercise'

Kimberley: How I work out with my kids

I've been working out with my kids since the twins were around seven months old. I actually stumbled upon the idea of involving them. I'd be outside doing some squats and one of the twins would become a little unsettled. Rather than stop, I'd just pick him up, raise him high, making sure I supported his neck and head, and off I went again. And they absolutely loved it! This technique never failed to turn a baby frown into a baby giggle, and it allowed me to fulfil my exercise goals.

When I was out walking with the kids in the pram I began to sneak in some lunges, rather than just walk. I'd sing to the babies while walking, lunging and walking – and it was a hit!

I decided to then explore the concept of involving the kids a little more, and I began to do push-ups off the pram and toe touches on the front wheel. Not only did the kids find it funny, but when I stopped they would start whingeing again. Talk about finding motivation and a cheering squad in places that I'd not thought to look. At times, when my energy was depleting, I had no choice but to keep going, because the babies were such tough coaches – and two laughing babies is always better than two crying babies any day.

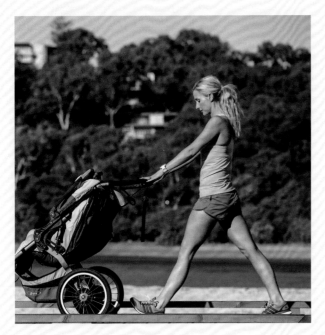

As the kids got older, they would walk around me, play or ride their bikes while I exercised. It just became part of our routine. As a mum, life was not always predictable, so I had to think outside the box and improvise when it came to finding new ways of incorporating some exercise into our everyday lives. The fitter I got, the more I actually enjoyed finding new ways to exercise with the kids in tow.

Be prepared

We all know that preparation is one of the crucial keys to maintaining sanity when you have kids. Having a routine and being well prepared can limit chaos and stress, and it's just the same when you're getting set to exercise.

If you want the kids to be entertained and let you do what you have to do, they'll need age-appropriate toys or items for entertainment, as well as food, drink and other essential items. If you have younger kids, you may need a play mat, comforters and hygiene items such as nappies and wipes to hand.

To maximise your organisation and preparation, it helps to have everything you'll need (and some you may not) all in one place and readily accessible, so that if you do need a quick break, you won't have to run around the house trying to find everything. If you have little ones, get your pram, bouncer, bike, scooter or other things to ensure they stay active, occupied and calm. Most little kids will also love to tinker with simple household items such as good old pots and pans from your kitchen. If it's hot, you can fill their play items with water and watch them stay cool while you get hot and sweaty.

Don't give in!

If things don't go quite as you planned when you're exercising with the kids in tow, don't quit. Stopping and starting is better than quitting. Realistically, the younger your kids are the more you'll have to stop and start and tend to the little ones, so just surrender to it and keep going. It is possible to do nappy changes, breastfeed and have complete outfit changes mid-workout. Sometimes it can even be considered a bonus to have to take a break in between. Once your kids get used to your daily routine (if you don't give in) they'll eventually let you do your thing for 15 minutes.

Create familiarity

To get your kids used to knowing when it's your time to exercise, it can help to stick to familiar times, days, objects and props. A great example of this would be to always use the same gym mat, clothing or room for your workout. With familiarity and routine, your kids will eventually come to know when its workout time, and they will even get to a stage where they'll know exactly what to expect. With encouragement and practice, they'll begin to get their pillows and toys, and whatever else they need to ready themselves, for a time that they know is dedicated to mummy enjoying some time to exercise. When you take a balanced and gentle approach to exercise, it's a wonderful thing for your children to see. Whenever our kids ask us why we are exercising, we always tell them it's because it makes us feel happy and strong.

Accept that sometimes it won't happen – without guilt

We've told you not to give in, but, as mums, we know that when kids come along, the best laid plans must sometimes be re-thought. On days when it really isn't working, or the kids are just too unsettled, you have to know that it is okay to let the workout slide. It's not the end of the world, and your sanity is worth more than one missed exercise routine. When this happens, it really is so important to give yourself a pat on the back for trying and just know that later in the afternoon or tomorrow might work better – for everyone. Lose the all-or-nothing approach and just accept that with young children not every day or everything goes to plan.

Encouraging exercise with teenagers

If you've got teenagers under your wing, whether they participate or not (could be a big ask), just keep in mind that they are still taking notice of what you are doing. When they see you consistently making healthy choices, they are going to eventually absorb that positive role modelling and potentially follow your example.

If your teenagers do join you on your quest for fitness, it's really important to consciously praise them for their efforts, even when you've had to drag them off the couch to do so. It might be of benefit to try alternative or more casual types of exercise if you want to involve the teens, such as walking, stair-run races, a skate-park expedition or a fun teenage workout with their friends. Friendly bribery never goes astray with kids too, so at the risk of our being a little cheeky, we highly recommend promising something you know they'll love if they participate, such as a big smoothie or another healthy treat once the mission is complete. They'll soon get hooked on the feeling that exercise and healthy eating brings if they participate often enough.

Five basic exercises for you and baby

Here are five staple exercises for you and baby. Please review the 'child-free' versions before beginning. (See pages 176–80 and 189)

Exercise musts when working out with baby

Once you're confident and have proper technique, it's great to involve your children in a workout whenever possible. Starting early when your child is just a baby is the perfect way to enhance your confidence, tone your body and start a healthy exercise routine. When exercising with your baby, it's important that he or she can independently hold their head up, even though you are supporting them.

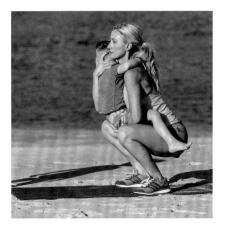

1. Squats

Hold your baby close and high up on your chest, with his head resting on your shoulder. Always make sure you support the back of your baby's neck and keep your chest high while looking up.

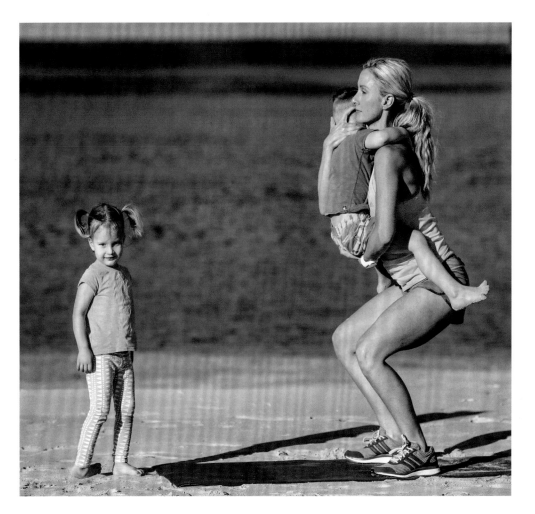

2. Lunges

If lunging with the pram, ensure that you are on a flat surface. Keep your arms relaxed, chest high and look forward, then drive off your front foot. If you're holding your baby, the same principles apply as when squatting.

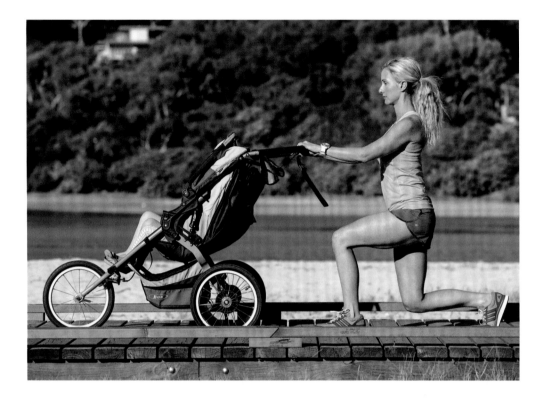

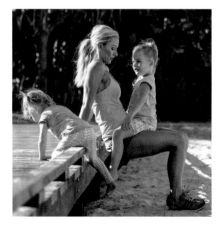

3. Dips

Place your baby in a secure position on your lap, if she is old enough, she can sit or lie on your chest. Ensure that you are in a seated position with your back and buttocks nice and close to the bench.

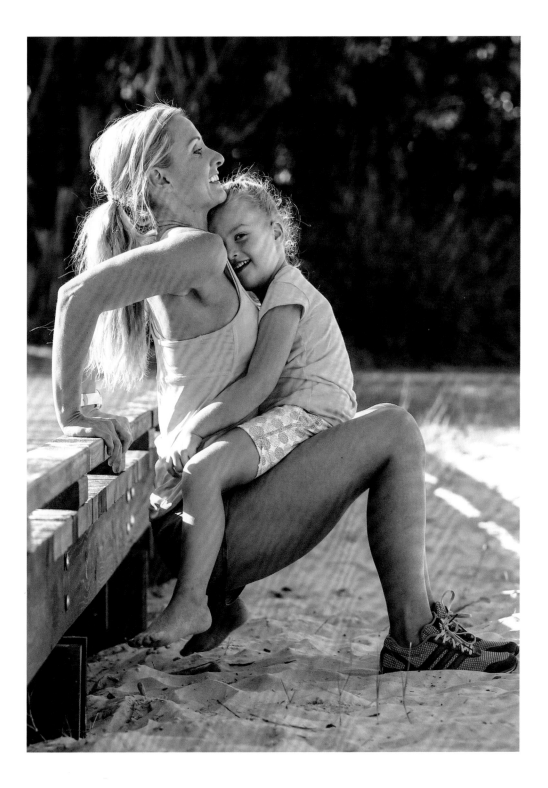

4. Push-ups

Lay your baby underneath you and in between your hands, then every time you lower yourself towards the ground, give your baby a kiss on the forehead.

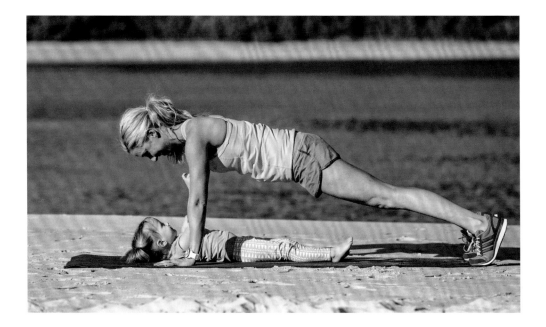

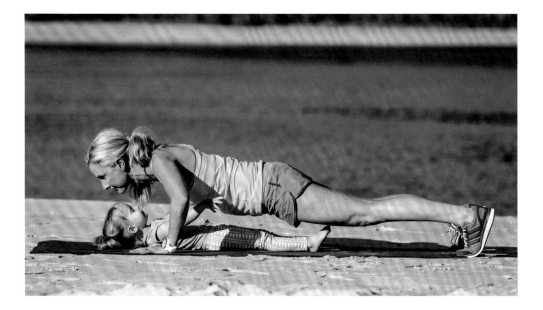

5. Mountain climbers

Lay your baby underneath you and in between your hands (in a push-up position) as you perform this exercise.

Start in a plank position, your hands a little wider than your shoulders. Alternately drive your knees forward, each time landing on the ball of your front foot. Alternate your legs while maintaining control through the trunk.

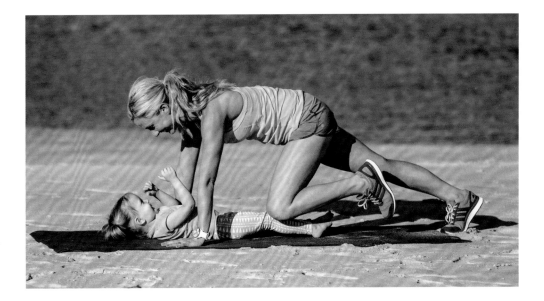

Common questions

Will I get bulky?

It's important to note that there are many young males in the gym who eat twice their body weight, take a mind-blowing 15 supplements per day and train seven days a week – yet they still have little to show for it. If being the beautiful female you are, training three or four times per week for 15 minutes and eating clean, nutrient-dense food turns you into a female Arnold, then let's bottle your genetics up now and sell it for millions to all those young men! Seriously, it's not going to happen. Under our routine and programme, and following our guidance, you will not turn into The Hulk. The main reason for bulk in women is generally because they are carrying too much body fat and it puts a layering on the muscle.

Bodyweight strength movements, or using weights, are very effective tools for providing load for our training. They can be used to stimulate many physiological changes in our bodies. Our primary reasons for strength work and using weights is to maintain or gain a little muscle (fat-burning furnace) and decrease our body fat.

Don't get swept up in the stigma of weights only being for bodybuilders. When we stretch, we are not scared of becoming contortionists, or when we're doing yoga, we're not concerned about becoming Buddhist monks. There is great value from using a little of all. We extract the best methods from many disciplines to be the most energised, mobile and strong women we can be.

Are there options for easier or harder workouts?

All the workouts in this Plan are adaptable for women from beginner to advanced fitness. Once you find your level of comfort with the movements, you can then up the intensity from there. If you need longer breaks, take them. If you can't get through all the rounds, get through most of them. If you can't get through the reps, set yourself a number and reach that instead. If you're comfortable with the movements and the Plan, then it's all about increasing the level of intensity that you are working at, or increasing the weights you are using for the strength work. Push yourself – these are shorter workouts but they are designed for you to get sweaty. Push for more reps and make every one count. If it doesn't challenge you it won't change you.

What if I have muscle separation or hernia?

We recommend seeing a post-natal physio before undertaking any level of exercise post-pregnancy.

What if I'm breastfeeding?

Yes, of course you can still workout if you are breastfeeding; however, based on our experience, we would recommend working out after a feed so that your breasts are soft and comfortable. Make sure you are wearing your breast pads, because we don't want that liquid gold flying everywhere. If you are breastfeeding, it is important to keep your energy levels up, especially when exercising. We would recommend having an extra smoothie or increasing your portion sizes to satisfy your hunger on the days that you work out.

What exercises are best for mummy tummy?

Tummy fat is just fat. Whether your fat is located on your hips, arms, legs or tummy, the solution is the same. The fitness industry has long debated the theory of 'spot reduction' and its existence. Spot reduction is the theory that you can shift fat from specific areas of the body and primarily about what exercise you use for those areas; for example, lie on the ground and do three sets of 50 sit-ups and a lactic-acid burn will fatigue you like never before. Fat loss is not specific to the working muscle area, however; in fact it's about overall energy expenditure.

More recently, however, science is softening on its lack of support for the spot-reduction theory, which proposes that specific exercises can be responsible for fat loss in target areas of our bodies. The larger movement exercises that transfer energy and movement through our mid-section at higher levels of intensity are shown to be up to 25 per cent more effective for reducing mummy tummies than other steady-state training methods (such as a 30-minute jog, bike ride or treadmill session). These larger movement exercises are the pillars of our programme.

Do I really need to use weights in my exercise programme?

Weights are simply an effective tool for applying resistance to a movement. Using weights in your exercise programme is not essential (they are optional) but by incorporating weights it allows you to measure resistance and overload movements easily and in a controlled and gradual manner, and they also assist in building added muscle.

If using weights really isn't for you, that's okay. If you are just starting out with weight use in your exercise programme, using your body weight (with no equipment) will still give you great results. If you are at more of an intermediate level and already know most of the movements, then it's great to use some light weights, such as dumbbells, for the workouts to build intensity and resistance. We recommend anywhere from 2kg to 10kg dumbbells, depending on your level of strength and experience.

If you are looking for a way to incorporate your kids into your daily workout, it's always fun to use them as weights – literally! And if the kids aren't interested in helping you exercise, you can use household items such as groceries (cans, filled plastic bottles) to increase the workout load. When your imagination is activated, your options are unlimited. And every time you pick up those grocery bags, canned foods or milk bottles, remember that they too make for the perfect weights in an impromptu two-minute workout!

Our end – is only the beginning

You've been drawn to this book for a reason. We know that you've felt the pull and you're ready to make some lasting changes to better yourself and your life. Whether you're an exhausted first-time mother clutching her precious newborn or an active mum that is just finding it harder and harder to get out that door, we know that Stay Strong Mummy can, and will, help you feel great and able to live the life you want.

If you're sick and tired of feeling flat, dull and carrying excess weight, if you've never exercised before or you're a full-time working mumma who just can't seem to get ahead, whoever you are and whatever your situation, this book is for you. And we are here for you too.

It's time, mumma. It's time for you to give yourself some tender loving care. It's time for you to focus on your own health and happiness. Your little people are watching your every move. We know that one of your greatest wishes for your children is for them to be healthy, but having happy, healthy kids begins with a happy and healthy mumma! Show your kids and everyone else just how healthy and happy mumma can be.

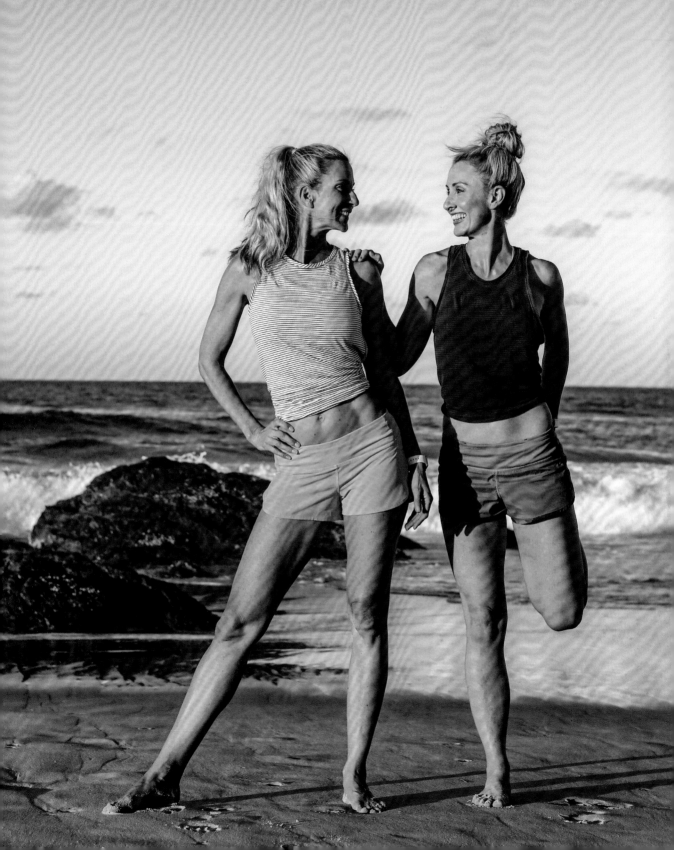

Index

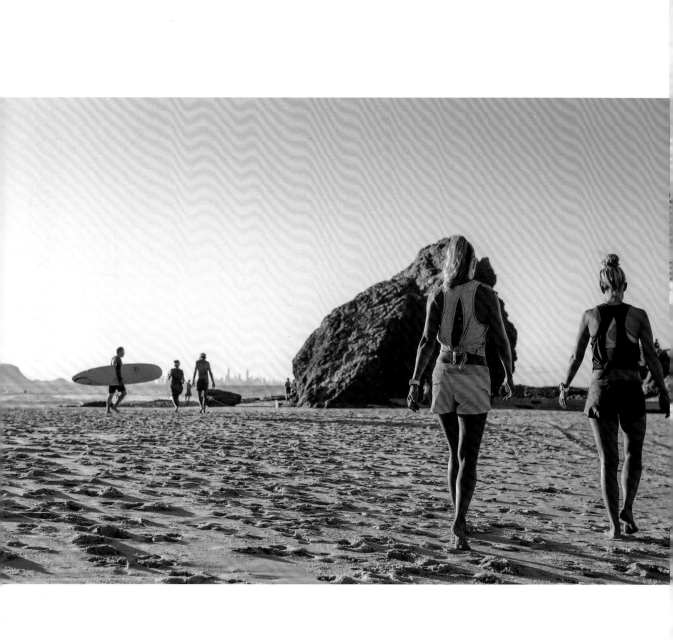